CLINICAL MANAGEMENT OF ADRENAL TUMORS

Edited by **John I. Lew**

Clinical Management of Adrenal Tumors
http://dx.doi.org/10.5772/63139
Edited by John I. Lew

Contributors

Marlon Guerrero Md, Vincenzo Neri, Ruth Prichard, Helen Heneghan, Alexandra Mirica, Diana Loreta Paun, Shivanshu Singh, Santosh Kumar, Luca Tajana, Antonio Osculati, Silvia Visonà, Tanya Castelino, Elliot Mitmaker, Tomaz Kocjan

Published by InTech
Janeza Trdine 9, 51000 Rijeka, Croatia

Publishing Process Manager Romina Skomersic
Technical Editor SPi Global
Cover InTech Design team

First published June, 2017
Printed in Croatia
Legal deposit, Croatia: National and University Library in Zagreb

Additional hard copies can be obtained from orders@intechopen.com

Clinical Management of Adrenal Tumors , Edited by John I. Lew
p. cm.
Print ISBN 978-953-51-3265-3
Online ISBN 978-953-51-3266-0

Meet the editor

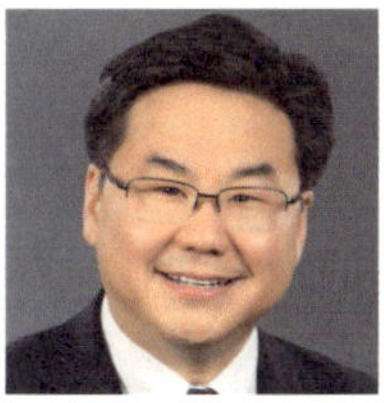

John I. Lew, MD, FACS, is an associate professor of Surgery and vice chair of Surgery of the DeWitt Daughtry Family Department of Surgery at the University of Miami Leonard M. Miller School of Medicine. He currently serves as the chief of the Division of Endocrine Surgery, fellowship director in Endocrine Surgery at the University of Miami/Jackson Memorial Hospitals, and physician leader of the Thyroid and Other Endocrine Cancer Site Disease Group at the University of Miami Sylvester Comprehensive Cancer Center. Dr. Lew is a nationally and internationally renowned endocrine surgeon for his clinical expertise that encompasses thyroid, parathyroid, and adrenal diseases. Dr. Lew's academic pursuits include surgical outcomes and translational research in the management of benign and malignant thyroid, parathyroid, and adrenal tumors. Dr. Lew has authored and coauthored numerous original papers in academic journals and several chapters in major textbooks in the field of endocrine and general surgery. He resides in Miami, Florida, with his wife and their two children.

Contents

Preface

Adrenal tumors are commonly encountered in the clinical setting most often discovered incidentally on imaging studies. Physicians in training and clinical practice will undoubtedly care for patients with adrenal tumors. With the aging population and widespread use of routine imaging, the incidence of patients with adrenal tumors is expected to continually increase in the years to come.

The clinical management of adrenal tumors has evolved over the last decade due to significant developments that include the identification of genetic alterations resulting in the pathogenesis of these tumors and the genotype and phenotype correlations that have clinical significance in their management. Further understanding and knowledge of these adrenal tumors with the advent of improved high-resolution imaging studies, advanced biochemical and genetic tests that help delineate between functional and nonfunctional adrenal tumors, and the evolution of highly developed surgical techniques and approaches have improved patient outcomes.

This book presents an overview of adrenal tumors written by a multidisciplinary team of world experts. It is not meant to be an all-encompassing treatise of adrenal tumors but rather focuses on current and timely subjects relevant in the clinical care of patients with adrenal tumors. Adrenal “incidentalomas" are initially discovered during cross imaging obtained for other clinical reasons. With advances in imaging and molecular histopathology over the past few years, unusual adrenal gland masses adrenal masses as a result of infection, benign tumors over the past few years have become better known. Recent and continued identification of gene mutations associated with pheochromocytomas and paragangliomas will ensure early diagnosis, prompt treatment, and better prognosis for patient and family members. Strong genetic determinism of pheochromocytomas and paragangliomas emphasizes the need for further studies to better understand the pathogenesis and malignant transformation of these particular tumors, which may have an important role in the development of future treatment options toward personalized therapy for patients.

Once thought rare, primary hyperaldosteronism is now considered the most common form of secondary hypertension among primary care and hypertensive patients. As the global burden of primary hyperaldosteronism is high, nal approach to patients with suspected primary hyperaldosteronism becomes warranted. Pheochromocytomas are rare catecholamine-secreting neuroendocrine tumors derived from chromaffin tissue of the adrenal medulla. Developments in the diagnosis of such most commonly benign hyperfunctioning adrenal tumors encompass biochemical, radiologic, histologic, and molecular analyses with novel therapeutic strategies and advances in individualized targeted therapies for the remaining rare malignant lesions. Pheochromocytoma multisystem crisis (PMC) is an uncommon rare and potential entity consisting of a tetrad of symptoms including hemodynamic instability and collapse, encephalopathy, hyperthermia, and multiorgan failure. Although its treatment remains controversial, there has been a paradigm shift in the surgical management of PMC, from performing emergency adrenalectomy immediately after the diagnosis to medical stabilization followed by elective adrenalectomy in more controlled and ideal situations.

Minimally invasive adrenalectomy is the preferred surgical treatment of adrenal tumors at many specialized medical centers worldwide with the choice of laparoscopic transabdominal or retroperitoneal approach strongly influenced by background training, skill, and experience of the surgeon. Two issues that constantly evolve with minimally invasive adrenalectomy are size limit of adrenal mass and appropriateness for malignant adrenal tumors. Rarely considered, but imperative for both clinicians and pathologists alike to consider these diseases in daily practice, the leading cause of sudden death related to adrenal gland disease is neuroendocrine tumor derived from chromaffin cells such as pheochromocytoma and paraganglioma, followed by adrenal hypofunction due to adrenal hemorrhage.

The book comprises a total of eight chapters from multiple contributors around the world, including Canada, India, Ireland, Italy, Romania, Slovenia, and the United States. The authors provide a comprehensive, art-based perspective of topics in their field, highlighting important relevant issues and trends. The book will serve as a valuable resource of information for medical students, residents in training, physicians, and researchers. I am grateful to all the contributors for the submission of their chapters in the preparation of this edited volume on clinical management of adrenal tumors. I hope this book will serve as a valuable source of information reference for all medical providers who care for tumors that are encountered in everyday practice and remain sometimes challenging to manage and decipher.

I express my gratitude to the InTech-Open Science Open Minds, the DeWitt Daughtry Family Department of Surgery, and the University of Miami Leonard M. Miller School of Medicine for their support in the task of publishing this volume. I remain grateful for the medical students, residents, and fellows in training who continue to teach and inspire me. I offer my thanks and appreciation to Ms. Romina Skomersic, Publishing Process Manager, for her patience and assistance in bringing out the book to its present form. I would also like to thank my teachers, mentors, and colleagues for their support. And finally, I would like to extend my special and heartfelt thanks to my wife, Alexandra, and my children, Mela Elisabeth and John Alexandre, for their unwavering love, patience, and support. I am indebted to all of the aforementioned for their invaluable help and assistance, but any errors or omissions that may remain herein are mine alone.

John I. Lew, MD, FACS
Division of Endocrine Surgery
DeWitt Daughtry Family Department of Surgery
University of Miami Leonard M. Miller School of Medicine,
Miami, USA

Chapter 1

Current Management of Adrenal Incidentalomas

Maria Michailidou and Marlon A. Guerrero

Additional information is available at the end of the chapter

http://dx.doi.org/10.5772/intechopen.68774

Abstract

Adrenal "incidentalomas" refer to a group of adrenal masses initially discovered during cross-sectional imaging obtained for other clinical reasons. The majority of incidentalomas are benign nonfunctional adrenal adenomas and can be safely managed expectantly. A subset of adrenal incidentalomas, however, are functional and/or malignant, and these lesions most often require adrenalectomy. The following chapter outlines the differential diagnosis, the different imaging modalities and features, as well as biochemical evaluation of adrenal incidentalomas.

Keywords: adrenal, mass, function

1. Introduction

An adrenal incidentaloma refers to an adrenal mass that is incidentally found on imaging studies not intended initially to assess the adrenal glands. This term does not include adrenal masses that were discovered in patients with a genetic predisposition to develop adrenal tumors nor in patients with extra-adrenal malignancies discovered on imaging studies for cancer staging purposes.

The frequency of adrenal incidentalomas varies in the literature. Autopsy studies report an incidence of adrenal incidentalomas ranging from 1 to 9% [1]. Frequency of adrenal incidentalomas reported in the radiology literature varies according to imaging modality. With computed tomography (CT) scans and magnetic resonance imaging (MRI), incidence of these adrenal tumors ranges from 0.3 to 7%, whereas prevalence of adrenal incidentalomas from ultrasound studies reaches 0.4–2% [2]. The discovery of adrenal incidentalomas increases with age where prevalence in patients <30 years of age is <1%, but 7% in patients >70 years of age. Furthermore, patients with obesity, diabetes, and hypertension are more likely to have an incidental adrenal masses [3].

2. Etiology

Adrenal incidentalomas are categorized by malignant potential and functionality. These categorizations are utilized to determine the necessity for surgical resection. Most adrenal incidentalomas are benign nonfunctioning adenomas (71%), but such lesions may represent lipomas, cysts, myelolipomas, hamartomas, ganglioneuromas, teratomas, neurofibromas, leiomyomatosis, hematomas, or infections. Malignant adrenal tumors are rare, consisting of primary adrenocortical carcinoma (4%) and metastases (2%) from other regions. Radiographic features and tumor size are used to predict the risk of malignancy.

Approximately 20% of functional adrenal incidentalomas, which occur less frequently than benign nonfunctional tumors, are found incidentally during imaging. Similarly, symptoms typical of adrenal hypersecretion are common in patients found to have hormonal syndromes, but functional adrenal incidentalomas are rarely symptomatic. Functional adrenal tumors include those that hypersecrete cortisol (8%), catecholamines (6%), and aldosterone (2%).

This chapter focuses on the comprehensive evaluation of incidental adrenal tumors (**Figure 1**). Classic imaging findings, clinical presentation, and surgical indications will also be outlined in detail.

2.1. Imaging characteristics

Although adrenal incidentalomas are found fortuitously on imaging, at times the features of these masses on imaging lend themselves to suggest a diagnosis (**Table 1**). The characteristics of adrenal tumors vary according to imaging modalities. Findings pertaining to specific imaging modalities are discussed further below.

Adrenal size is one of the most important determinants of malignancy. Prior guidelines recommended adrenalectomy for patients with an adrenal mass ≥6 cm [4, 5]. However, in one of the largest multicenter retrospective studies, adrenal tumor size >4 cm provided the highest sensitivity (93%) in differentiating between benignity and malignancy [6]. The authors also showed that adrenocortical carcinoma (ACC) was more common in younger patients compared to those patients with benign adenomas (median age 46 years versus 57 years). Due to the aggressive nature and rapid growth rate of ACC, and since achieving free margins is one of the most important determinants in extending patient survival [6, 7], current guidelines suggest adrenalectomy in all surgically fit patients with an adrenal mass >4 cm [8, 9].

2.1.1. Computed tomography

Specific tumor characteristics on computed tomography (CT) help differentiate benign from malignant adrenal tumors. The majority of benign adrenal adenomas has a high intracellular

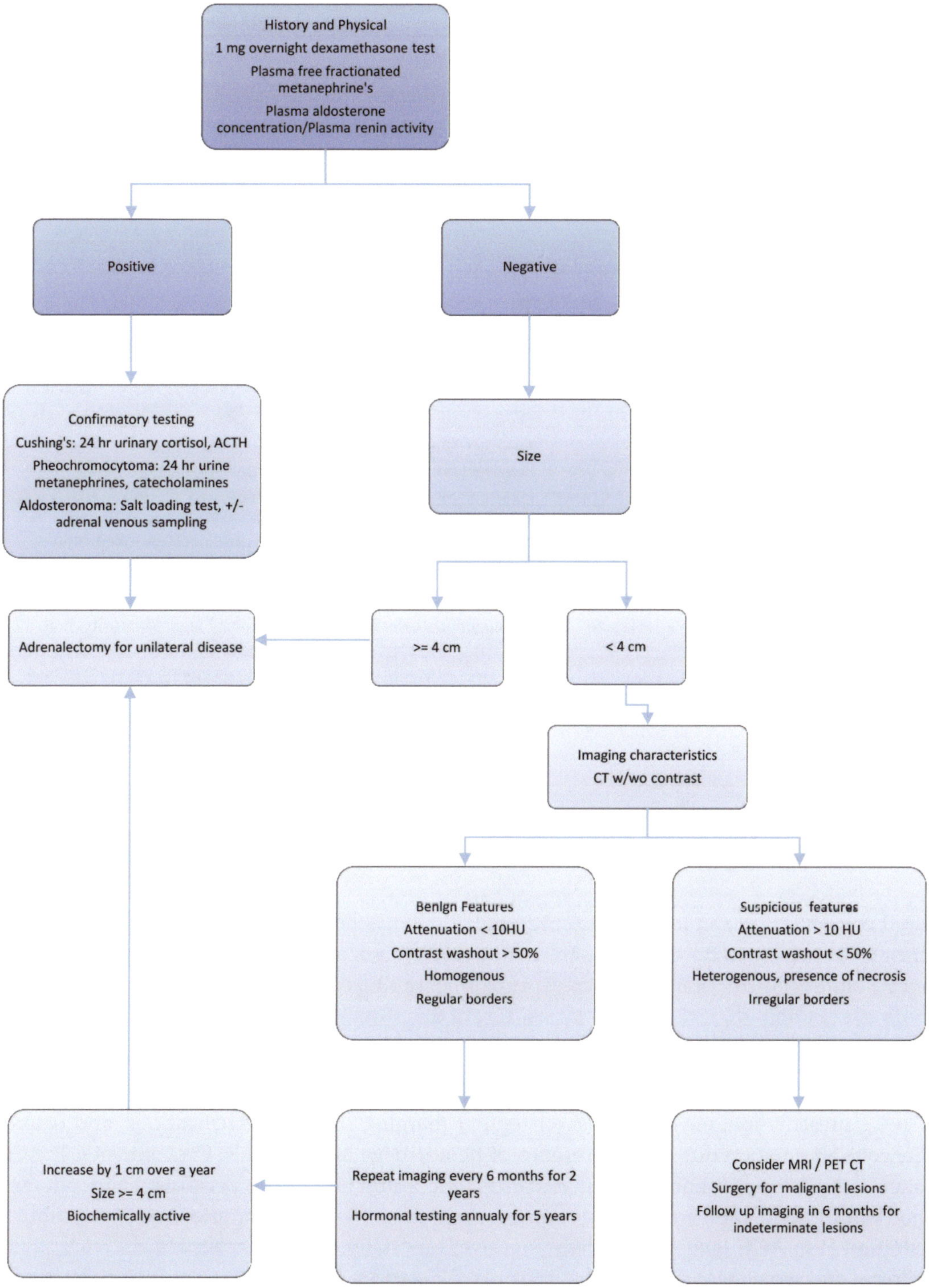

Figure 1. Work-up algorithm of a solitary adrenal incidentaloma.

Adrenal masses	Average size	CT findings	MRI findings
Lipid-rich adenoma	<4 cm	Well circumscribed, homogenous, <10 HU on unenhanced CT, >60% absolute contrast washout, >40% relative contrast washout	Homogenous intermediate T1 signal intensity, low T2 signal intensity, loss of signal at out-of-phase images
Lipid-poor adrenal adenoma	<4 cm	Well circumscribed, homogenous, >10 HU on unenhanced CT, >60% absolute contrast washout, >40% relative contrast washout	Homogenous, intermediate T1 signal intensity, lack of signal loss at out-of-phase images
Adrenocortical carcinoma	≥4 cm	Irregular, inhomogenous, >10 HU on unenhanced CT, <60% absolute contrast washout, <40% relative contrast washout	Low T1 heterogeneous signal High T2 signal intensity with nonenhancing necrotic components, lack of signal loss on out-of-phase images
Pheochromocytoma	2–5 cm	Irregular, with calcifications, heterogeneous, > 10 HU on unenhanced CT, avid enhancement due to hypervascularity	Inhomogenous, low T1 signal intensity, high T2 signal intensity ("light bulb sign"), thick enhancing wall with central necrosis, calcifications, lack of signal loss on out-of-phase images
Metastatic lesion	Variable size	Homogenous/heterogeneous based on size, irregular, >10 HU, <60% absolute contrast washout, <40% relative contrast washout, increase in size on interval imaging, unilateral versus bilateral	Low T1 signal intensity, high T2 signal intensity, heterogeneous enhancement, presence or lack of signal loss on out-of-phase images depending on presence of intracytoplasmic lipid

Table 1. Typical computed tomography (CT) scan and magnetic resonance imaging (MRI) findings for individual adrenal masses.

lipid concentration and low density. Adrenal adenomas possess low attenuation on noncontrast CT represented by <10 hounsfield units (HU) (**Figure 2**). However, density alone is not an absolute predictor of malignancy. Approximately 30% of adenomas have low lipid content with attenuation >10 HU on noncontrast CT. In this situation, intravenous contrast enhancement may be helpful. Benign adrenal adenomas usually have a density of 80–90 HU with IV contrast, and a >50% washout on delayed images.

On CT presentation, most ACC have irregular margins, irregular calcifications, and heterogeneous attenuation due to the presence of hemorrhage and necrosis. On contrast CT, ACC often demonstrates inhomogenous enhancement, a thin enhancing peripheral rim, attenuation value >10 HU, and an absolute contrast washout <60% after 15 minutes of contrast administration [10]. ACC tend to be locally invasive, especially in vascular structures such as the adrenal and renal veins, and inferior vena cava. However, imaging alone cannot discriminate functioning from nonfunctioning adenomas. Although some radiographic findings may suggest a diagnosis, functionality of adrenal tumors is made biochemically.

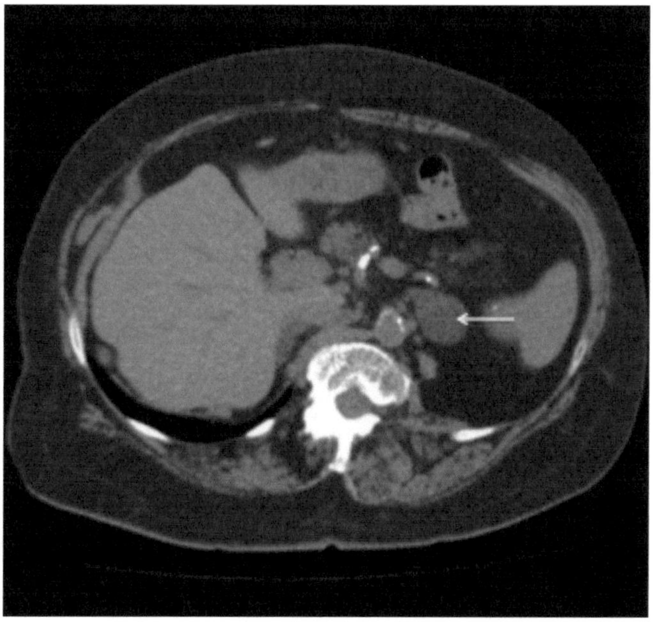

Figure 2. A 72-year-old female with 2.6 cm low-attenuating homogenous left adrenal mass (arrow) on noncontrast CT of the abdomen consistent for adrenal adenoma.

On noncontrast CT, majority of pheochromocytomas are well-circumscribed, round-to-oval masses with peripheral calcifications. Size varies (average 5 cm), but due to presence of necrosis and/or hemorrhage, pheochromocytomas demonstrate heterogeneous attenuation. With contrast enhancement, pheochromocytomas display heterogeneous enhancement, density >100 HU, and retention of contrast on delayed imaging.

Other functioning adrenal tumors do not have specific CT characteristics that are definitive for diagnosis, but there are some general features that should be kept in mind. Cortisol-secreting adrenal adenomas are usually small (average: 2–2.5 cm), and low-density lesions due to its high lipid concentration. Similarly, most aldosteronomas are <2 cm, solitary, and eccentric within the adrenal gland. However, the majority of patients with hyperaldosteronism has bilateral hyperplasia and, therefore, require adrenal venous sampling to help identify a unilateral adenoma, even when finding a single adenoma on imaging.

Benign adrenal cysts are homogenous, nonenhancing lesions with attenuation near that of water (8 HU). Cysts may develop with or without wall calcifications, but the wall of the cyst is consistently <3 mm. Myelolipomas are rare benign tumors composed of bone marrow elements. These tumors vary in size, but measure on average 5 cm. Their radiographic appearance depends on their histological composition, but the presence of local macroscopic fat is diagnostic in all cases (**Figure 3**). Fat-rich myelolipomas have unenhanced attenuation typically between −50 and −100 HU. They contain a pseudocapsule and about 20% have calcifications, especially when prior hemorrhage has occurred. Adrenal hematomas can be unilateral or bilateral, and typically have unenhanced attenuation values of 55–90 HU.

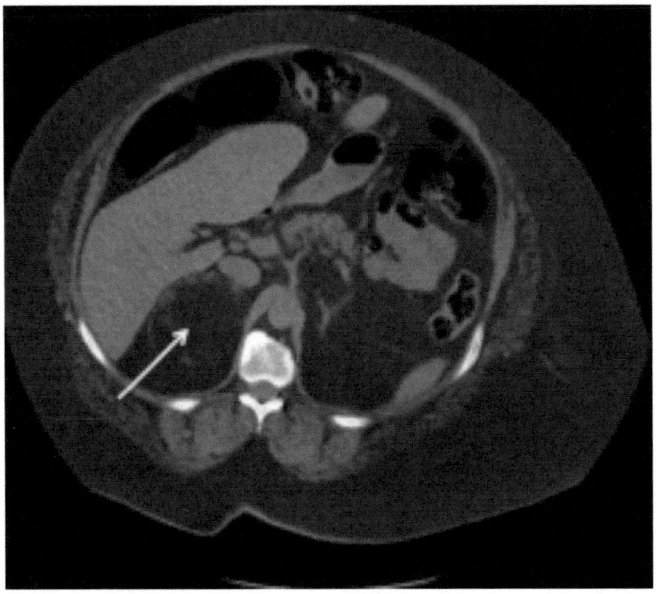

Figure 3. A 55-year-old female with 7.7 cm fat—containing right adrenal mass (arrow) on noncontrast CT of the abdomen. Surgical pathology consistent for myelolipoma.

2.1.2. Magnetic resonance imaging

Recent advances in technology that have made magnetic resonance imaging (MRI) prominent in the imaging of adrenal tumors include gradient-echo breath-hold scans, chemical shift imaging with in-phase and out-of-phase T1-weighted sequences to detect intracellular lipid and water protons, as well as three-dimensional dynamic imaging.

Chemical shift MRI is based on differences in the frequencies the protons in water and fat display within a magnetic field. During in-phase imaging, the signals of water and fat protons are additive, whereas during out-of-phase imaging their signals are subtracted. Therefore, lipid-rich adenomas show loss of signal on out-of-phase imaging, while lipid-poor adenomas display modest signal loss. In equivocal cases, a relative drop in signal compared with the spleen establishes the presence of microscopic fat to help differentiate adenomas [11]. Benign adrenal adenomas are usually iso- or hypointense on T2 weighted images. Adenomas also present with early peak homogenous enhancement (usually within 52 seconds), which helps discriminate fat poor adenomas from malignant masses.

Pheochromocytoma has a typical appearance on MRI. These functional tumors usually present with increased T2 signal intensity compared to adenomas, and in <50% of cases display the classic "light-bulb bright" T2 appearance (**Figure 4**). T2 hyperintensity is due to high fluid content and hypervascularity. In addition, the absence of microscopic fat results in absent signal loss between the in- and out-of-phase images. Adrenal masses with these findings are highly suggestive of pheochromocytoma, but lipid poor ACC or adrenal metastatic lesions may also have similar MRI characteristics.

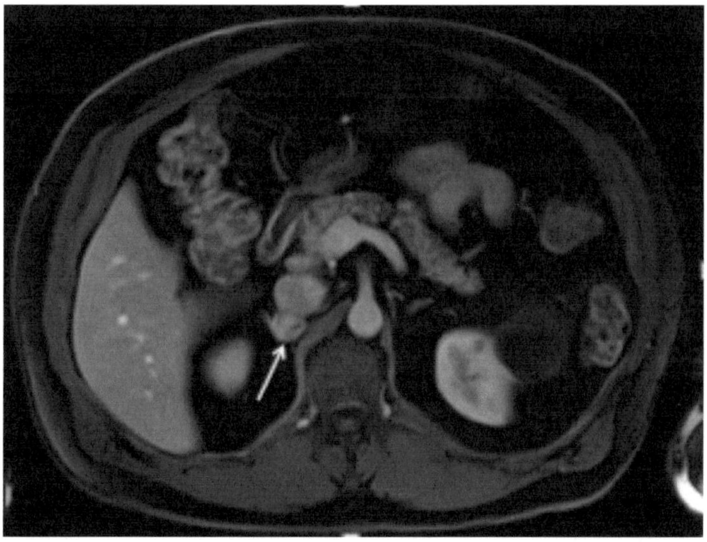

Figure 4. A 62-year-old male with biochemically confirmed pheochromocytoma. MRI abdomen demonstrating 1.7 cm right adrenal mass (arrow) with markedly enhanced heterogeneous T2 signal typical of pheochromocytoma.

As with CT scan, MRI cannot accurately differentiate functional adrenal masses. MRI shows similar sensitivity and specificity with CT in recognizing aldosteronomas. However, bilateral adrenal hyperplasia and unilateral aldosterone-producing adenomas show similar signal loss during out-of-phase sequences. Patients with adrenal Cushing's syndrome will display MRI findings consistent for a lipid-rich adenoma. In some cases, indirect findings of a unilateral cortisol-producing adenoma include atrophy of the nonadenomatous contralateral adrenal gland due to suppressed stimulation from Adrenocorticotropic hormone (ACTH).

Some nonfunctioning adrenal masses have certain identifiable features on MRI. For instance, benign adrenal cysts appear as hypointense lesions on T1-weighted images and hyperintense lesions with a hypointense rim on T2-weighted images. The presence of macroscopic fat within myelolipomas yields a distinctive high T1 and moderate T2 signal intensity, with loss of signal of fat saturation in out-of-phase chemical shift sequences.

Adrenal hematoma has three distinct characteristics depending on their time of imaging. Acute (<7 days) adrenal hematoma will appear iso- or hypointense on T1-weighted images and markedly hypointense on T2-weighted images. Subacute (1 week to 2 months) hematoma will appear hyperintense on T1-weighted images. In the chronic stage (2–3 months), a T2-hypointense rim will appear along the periphery of the adrenal hematoma secondary to hemosiderin-laden macrophages.

For ACC, T1 sequences display a low heterogeneous signal, whereas on T2-weighted images, they appear hyperintense with nonenhancing necrotic components. Additionally, multiplanar MRI images allow identification of adrenal tissue when the tumor is invading into adjacent structures and the origin of the tumor cannot be distinguished.

2.1.3. Positron emission tomography (PET)

Normally functioning adrenal glands are usually not fluorodeoxyglucose (FDG) avid. FDG positron emission tomography (PET) allows the evaluation of primary lesions and metastases with excellent sensitivities. By definition, an adrenal mass found during cancer surveillance or staging does not constitute an adrenal incidentaloma. However, adrenal masses can be found incidentally in PET scan conducted for other reasons besides cancer surveillance or staging.

The evaluation of adrenal glands with FDG PET usually originates from its use in lung cancer staging. An adrenal lesion is considered malignant if it typically displays higher Standardized Uptake Values (SUV) values than the liver (1.5). However, a recent study reported 99% sensitivity and 92% specificity of PET CT in differentiating benign from malignant adrenal lesions when a cut-off value of SUV_{max} of 3.1 was used. According to recent meta-analysis, mean sensitivity, specificity, positive likelihood ratio, negative likelihood ratio, and diagnostic odds ratio values for differentiating between benign and malignant adrenal disease were 0.97 (95% CI: 0.93, 0.98), 0.91 (95% CI: 0.87, 0.94), 11.1 (95% CI: 7.5, 16.3), 0.04 (95% CI: 0.02, 0.08), and 294 (95% CI: 107, 805), respectively [12]. Another study showed 100% sensitivity and 88% specificity in distinguishing ACC from adrenal adenoma, when a cut-off value of above 1.45 for adrenal-to-liver SUV_{max} ratio was used [13]. False-positive results, however, may arise in patients with pheochromocytoma, adrenal hyperplasia, and functioning adenomas (5%).

Currently, routine use of PET CT in the evaluation of adrenal incidentalomas has not been validated, and it is primarily used in patients with prior history of malignancy with nondiagnostic findings on CT scan.

2.2. Presentation and biochemical testing of functional adrenal tumors

Hormonal evaluation of adrenal incidentalomas is paramount for proper evaluation and diagnosis. Despite advances in imaging technology, no radiographic finding can definitively establish a diagnosis without biochemical testing. In this section, the appropriate biochemical testing for an adrenal incidentaloma is described.

2.2.1. Hypercortisolism

The most common cause of hypercortisolism is exogenous glucocorticoid use. Of the endogenous causes, most affected individuals (75%) will have Cushing's disease caused by an ACTH-secreting pituitary adenoma. The remainder is composed of cortisol-secreting adrenal adenomas (15%) and ectopic ACTH syndrome (<10%), usually caused by neuroendocrine tumors or bronchogenic malignant neoplasms arising in the thoracic cavity. Patients with hypercortisolism present with a variety of signs and manifestations; however, those subset of patients with adrenal incidentalomas are rarely symptomatic. Signs and symptoms of adrenal Cushing's syndrome include central obesity, moon facies, purple striae, hypertension, easy bruising, plethora, hirsutism, muscle weakness, glucose intolerance or diabetes, osteopenia, menstrual irregularities, and emotional disturbances. More commonly, patients with adrenal incidentalomas present as subclinical Cushing syndrome, with no findings suggestive of hypercortisolism.

Three screening tests are commonly used to make the diagnosis of hypercortisolism and are based on several pathophysiological derangements. First, excess cortisol secretion can be detected by an elevated 24 hours urine-free cortisol with the diagnosis made when cortisol is four times the normal value. Loss of normal diurnal cortisol variation is best detected by testing late-night salivary cortisol between 11 pm and midnight, and a value >2.0 ng/mL is diagnostic. Second, loss of negative feedback is best detected with a low-dose dexamethasone suppression test where 1 mg of dexamethasone is given at 11 pm and serum cortisol is tested at 8 am the next morning. Suppression of cortisol level <1.8 μg/dL has the best negative predictive value for Cushing's disease. Diagnosis of subclinical Cushing's syndrome is confirmed with a serum cortisol level ≥5.0 μg/dL after a 1 mg dexamethasone suppression test [9]. Finally, after diagnosis has been established, ACTH levels will further determine if the cause of hypercortisolism originates in the pituitary or adrenal glands. Undetectable ACTH levels are consistent with adrenal origin. In patients with high ACTH levels, a combination of brain MRI, high-dose dexamethasone suppression test, and bilateral petrosal sinus ACTH sampling will determine the origin of ACTH production and further guide appropriate treatment.

2.2.2. *Pheochromocytoma*

Pheochromocytoma refers to a tumor of catecholamine producing cells, the majority of which arise in the adrenal medulla and affects about 0.2% of hypertensive individuals. A small percentage (1–2%), known as paragangliomas, arise from chromaffin-producing neural crest cells that parallel the sympathetic and parasympathetic ganglia. These locations include the para-aortic sympathetic chain, the sympathetic and parasympathetic chain of the neck, posterior mediastinum, and the organ of Zuckerkandl. The hallmark of pheochromocytoma is persistent hypertension with episodic headaches, sweating, and tachycardia. Other common symptoms of this disease include palpitations, orthostatic hypotension, heart disease, pallor, nausea, anxiety, and flushing. Approximately 10% of patients, however, remain asymptomatic.

Most pheochromocytomas secrete norepinephrine, epinephrine, and rarely dopamine. Traditionally, diagnosis was based on 24 hours measurement of urine catecholamines and metanephrines. Plasma-free metanephrines are produced continuously through metabolism of catecholamines within pheochromocytoma tumor cells, in contrast to episodic secretion of catecholamines [14]. Plasma metanephrine levels exceeding 3–4 times normal are highly diagnostic for pheochromocytoma (normal value <0.5 nmol/L). Given the rarity of pheochromocytomas, and 86% specificity observed with plasma-free metanephrine tests, confirmation needs to be established with measurement of 24 hours urine metanephrines and catecholamines. In equivocal cases, clonidine suppression test may be obtained, which measures plasma-free metanephrines after oral administration of 0.3 mg of clonidine. It is important to discontinue medications such as phenoxybenzamine, sympathomimetics, acetaminophen, and tricyclic antidepressants prior to any biochemical testing due to interference with the results.

Patients with concerns for metastatic disease due to large size of primary tumor or extra-adrenal, multifocal, or suspected genetic components, should undergo ^{123}I meta-iodobenzylguanidine (MIBG) scintigraphy. PET CT is the preferred imaging modality over MIBG scan in patients with metastatic disease. Up to 25% of pheochromocytomas occur in the setting of hereditary syndrome, such as multiple endocrine neoplasia types 2A and B, von Hippel-Lindau disease, neurofibromatosis type 1, and hereditary paraganglioma syndrome. Therefore, genetic testing needs to be obtained in a subset of patients less than 50 years, with bilateral or multifocal disease or malignant extra-adrenal disease.

2.2.3. *Primary hyperaldosteronism*

Primary hyperaldosteronism (Conn's syndrome) is the most common cause of secondary hypertension, and it refers to a group of disorders in which aldosterone production by the zona glomerulosa is inappropriately high, relatively autonomous, and independent of the renin-angiotensin system. The most common cause of primary hyperaldosteronism is bilateral adrenal hyperplasia (60%), followed by functional unilateral adenoma (35%), unilateral adrenal hyperplasia (2%), and rarely functional adrenocortical carcinoma (1%), ectopic aldosterone producing tumor (1%), and familiar hyperaldosteronism (1%).

Most patients with primary hyperaldosteronism are asymptomatic, but all have hypertension. Hypertension associated with Conn's syndrome is unique in that it is not only persistent but also progressive and difficult to control. Patients with primary hyperaldosteronism usually require multiple hypertensive medications, often are taking more than three. Patients with an adrenal incidentaloma without hypertension do not have Conn's syndrome, and do not need to undergo biochemical testing for primary hyperaldosteronism. Furthermore, the pathognomonic finding of hypertension and hypokalemia is highly suggestive of Conn's syndrome, but only 30% present in this manner. Symptoms associated with hypokalemia are muscle weakness, polyuria, polydipsia, nocturia due to nephrogenic diabetes insipidus, paresthesias, and, rarely, tetany.

The most reliable screening method for primary hyperaldosteronism is the ratio of plasma aldosterone concentration (PAC) to plasma renin activity (PRA). Screening should be performed by taking a random morning PAC and PRA value after correction of hypokalemia due to interference with aldosterone secretion. Aldosterone receptor antagonists spironolactone and eplerenone, as well as high-dose amiloride, are the only medications that absolutely affect the interpretation of the PAC:PRA ratio, and these medications should be discontinued 5–6 weeks before the screening test. A PAC:PRA ratio ≥20 along with a PAC value ≥15 ng/ml is considered a positive test for primary aldosteronism. Given the negative feedback on renin, PRA is suppressed in Conn's syndrome, and an elevated PRA excludes the diagnosis. A confirmation salt loading test may be performed following a positive screening test, or in patients with equivocal results. Typically, a three-day oral salt loading test (>200 mEq/day) is performed and 24 hours urine aldosterone excretion is measured. A urine aldosterone excretion ≥12 μg/24 hours confirms primary hyperaldosteronism. Alternatively, PAC is measured after intravenous infusion of 2 L of normal saline over 4 hours. A PAC value ≥10 ng/dL supports the diagnosis.

Following biochemical diagnosis of primary hyperaldosteronism, adrenal venous sampling (AVS) should be performed to differentiate unilateral adenoma from bilateral hyperplasia. All patients found to have an adrenal mass <1 cm require AVS. Unfortunately, there is a lack of standardized protocols, and therefore, the procedure as well as interpretation of results can vary between medical centers [15]. AVS requires sampling of bilateral adrenal veins and peripheral (inferior vena cava) locations for aldosterone and cortisol. Cortisol is utilized to confirm successful cannulation of the adrenal veins. A more than fivefold elevation of the cortisol concentration in the adrenal vein sample relative to peripheral blood is confirmatory, and it is referred as the selectivity index. The side of aldosterone secretion is determined by the lateralization index that compares the aldosterone to cortisol ratios of the dominant to nondominant side. A ratio greater than 4:1 confirms unilateral adenoma and surgery should be considered. Some centers advocate the use of cosyntropin (either as continuous or bolus infusion) when performing AVS, especially when baseline successful cannulation rates are low. One study found a significant increase in the selectivity index after ACTH infusion; however, no effects were observed on the lateralization index [16]. Overall, when performed correctly, adrenal vein sampling has a sensitivity of 95% and specificity of 100% in detecting unilateral autonomous aldosterone secretion.

2.2.4. *Adrenocortical carcinoma*

Adrenocortical carcinoma (ACC) is a rare tumor and carries poor prognosis. At time of diagnosis, the majority are very large in size (mean size 9–13 cm), extend beyond the adrenal gland and metastatic. About two-thirds of all ACC are hormonally active and manifest with hypercortisolism and virilization and rarely hyperaldosteronism and feminization. About 20% of ACC will display virilization, whereas about one-fourth of cases will present with a mixed picture of Cushing's syndrome and virilization. However, when discovered as adrenal incidentalomas, they tend to be clinically biochemical inactive. Some patients may present with flank pain, abdominal discomfort, or fever due to hemorrhage within the tumor. All patients with radiographically suspected ACC, even when asymptomatic, should undergo biochemical evaluation for Cushing's syndrome, hyperaldosteronism, and be tested for sex steroids and its precursors (androstenedione, testosterone, dehydroepiandrosterone sulfate, and 17β-estradiol in postmenopausal women and men only). Identification of biochemical markers does not only aid in the perioperative management, but hormonal markers serve as tumor markers during postoperative surveillance.

2.2.5. *Other rare tumors (sex steroid-producing tumors)*

Sex steroid-producing tumors are rare. Most of these tumors are virilizing and may manifest at a late stage in association with an advanced ACC. Almost all feminizing tumors are malignant, whereas one-third of virilizing tumors are malignant.

2.3. Surgical indications and preoperative preparation

2.3.1. *Hypercortisolism*

Patients with unilateral cortisol-producing adenoma will have resolution of symptoms in about 90% of cases when treated surgically. Resolution of symptoms may take months to years to occur. Certain clinical manifestations, such as bone density, body composition, and inflammation may be persistent. Given the progressive negative systemic effect of hypercortisolism, patients with Cushing's syndrome should undergo adrenalectomy. Studies have also shown that patients with subclinical Cushing's syndrome may also benefit from adrenalectomy. A randomized study comparing adrenalectomy over medical management in patients with subclinical Cushing's syndrome showed that in the surgical group, diabetes mellitus normalized or improved in 63% of patients, hypertension in 67%, hyperlipidaemia in 38%, and obesity in 50%, whereas some patients in the medical group showed worsening of those parameters [17].

Patients with unilateral adrenal Cushing's syndrome will have chronic hypothalamic-pituitary-adrenal (HPA) axis suppression. As a result, the contralateral adrenal gland displays atrophy that is resistant to ACTH stimulation. Therefore, perioperative and postoperative corticosteroids need to be administered. Glucocorticoid administration needs to be continued on average 6–18 months until the HPA axis has completely recovered.

2.3.2. *Pheochromocytoma*

All patients with pheochromocytomas should undergo surgical resection. Laparoscopic adrenalectomy is commonly the treatment of choice. Tumors that suggest malignancy, such as large lesions, or those with evidence of local tumor invasion, should be resected with an open approach to avoid capsule disruption or tumor seeding. Cortical-sparing adrenalectomy is recommended in patients with hereditary pheochromocytoma, with small tumors and prior history of contralateral adrenalectomy in order to prevent permanent adrenal insufficiency.

After pheochromocytoma localization by imaging, all patients need to be started on α-blocker to counteract the sympathetic effects of catecholamine-producing cells. Goal of medical treatment should aim at reversing the downregulation of α-adrenergic receptors, and therefore, prevent intraoperative hemodynamic instability after tumor removal. Treatment should be initiated for at least 2 weeks preoperatively with the goal of eliciting orthostatic hypotension. The most frequently used alpha agent is phenoxybenzamine, which constitutes a nonselective, irreversible $\alpha 1$ agent with the longest half-life. Medical treatment is started at 10 mg twice daily, and titrated up to 300–400 mg daily until the patient becomes normotensive or develops intolerable side effects. Alternative agents include prazosin and terazosin. β-blockers, preferably propranolol, should be added in patients who develop persistent tachycardia or arrhythmias when α-blockade is initiated.

Intraoperatively, close communication between surgeon and anesthesiologist is essential. Invasive monitoring is mandated, and α and β-blocking agents as well as vasopressors need to be readily available. Excessive surgical manipulation of the tumor should be avoided, as it can stimulate further catecholamine secretion. Postoperatively, all patients need to be closely monitored for hypotension and hypoglycemia. Antihypertensive agents, with the exception of β-blockers, should be withheld and only used in patients with underlying essential hypertension. Patients with incomplete tumor removal or known metastatic disease should continue the use of α-blockers. Postoperatively, all patients need lifelong yearly follow-up for risk of recurrence.

2.3.3. *Primary hyperaldosteronism*

Patients with a unilateral aldosterone-producing adenoma commonly undergo laparoscopic adrenalectomy. Excess plasma aldosterone levels are deleterious, even when hypertension and hypokalemia are adequately controlled. Long-term sequelae of aldosterone excess include myocardial fibrosis, left ventricular hypertrophy, congestive heart failure, myocardial infarction, and stroke. Reductions in blood pressure and number of antihypertensive medications, as well as plasma and urine aldosterone levels can be observed as soon as 24 hours after successful surgery. Hypokalemia will resolve in all cases, whereas more than 80% of patients will show significant improvement of hypertension. Between 30 and 60% of patients will be completely weaned off antihypertensive medications, especially the young population with a short clinical course.

The following subset of patients show reduced benefit from adrenalectomy and will continue to require antihypertensive medications postoperatively: patients with a prolonged clinical course, men >45 years old, patients nonresponsive to spironolactone, need for more than two antihypertensive medications, and positive family history of hypertension. Patients with a delay in diagnosis often have irreversible secondary cardiovascular and renal changes rendering adrenalectomy less effective.

2.3.4. *Adrenocortical carcinoma*

Patients with radiographically suspected ACC who are surgically fit should undergo open adrenalectomy. The following concerning CT features indicate malignancy: unenhanced attenuation >10 HU, tumor >4 cm, irregular margins, nonhomogenous contrast enhancement, or local invasion to adjacent structures, especially the inferior vena cava. In cases of local invasion of adjacent structures, *en bloc* resection of the adrenal gland with the involved organ should be performed. Capsule disruption should be avoided, since it increases local recurrence. Traditionally, if ACC was recognized intraoperatively, conversion to an open procedure was mandated, since the laparoscopic approach had been linked to increased local recurrence, tumor seeding at port sites, and peritoneal spread. A recent study, however, has shown no difference in long-term oncological outcomes in carefully selected patients with stage I/II ACC, tumors <10 cm, and no evidence of extra-adrenal invasion, who underwent laparoscopic adrenalectomy by experienced surgeons [18].

2.4. Follow-up for nonoperative patients

Patients with adrenal incidentalomas who do not fulfill criteria for surgical resection should undergo repeat imaging at 3–6 months, and then annually, for 1–2 years. In addition, hormonal evaluation should be obtained annually for 5 years. The risk of enlargement during 1, 2, and 5 years is 6, 14, and 29%, respectively, and the risk of the mass becoming hormonally active during the same periods is 17, 29, and 47%, respectively. The most common hormonally active lesion in patients with previously inactive adenomas is subclinical Cushing's syndrome. Indications for surgical resection during follow-up include conversion to functional tumor and enlargement over 1 cm during follow-up imaging.

3. Summary

The majority of adrenal incidentalomas represent nonfunctioning adenomas. Unique imaging features of an adrenal mass, along with appropriate history and biochemical evaluation, can help determine the underlying diagnosis for adrenal incidentalomas and guide further treatment. Patients who do not fulfill surgical criteria should undergo repeat imaging as well as biochemical evaluation and expectant management.

Author details

Maria Michailidou and Marlon A. Guerrero*

*Address all correspondence to: mguerrero@surgery.arizona.edu

Department of Surgery, Banner University Medical Center Tucson, AZ, USA

References

[1] Terzolo M, Stigliano A, Chiodini I, Loli P, Furlani L, Arnaldi G, et al. AME position statement on adrenal incidentaloma. European Journal of Endocrinology/European Federation of Endocrine Societies. 2011;**164**(6):851-870

[2] Aron D, Terzolo M, Cawood TJ. Adrenal incidentalomas. Best Practice & Research Clinical Endocrinology & Metabolism. 2012;**26**(1):69-82

[3] Barzon L, Sonino N, Fallo F, Palu G, Boscaro M. Prevalence and natural history of adrenal incidentalomas. European Journal of Endocrinology/European Federation of Endocrine Societies. 2003;**149**(4):273-285

[4] Ross NS, Aron DC. Hormonal evaluation of the patient with an incidentally discovered adrenal mass. The New England Journal of Medicine. 1990;**323**(20):1401-1405

[5] NIH state-of-the-science statement on management of the clinically inapparent adrenal mass ("incidentaloma"). NIH Consensus and State-of-the-Science Statements. 2002;**19**(2):1-25

[6] Mantero F, Terzolo M, Arnaldi G, Osella G, Masini AM, Ali A, et al. A survey on adrenal incidentaloma in Italy. Study group on adrenal tumors of the Italian Society of Endocrinology. The Journal of Clinical Endocrinology and Metabolism. 2000;**85**(2):637-644

[7] Kim Y, Margonis GA, Prescott JD, Tran TB, Postlewait LM, Maithel SK, et al. Nomograms to predict recurrence-free and overall survival after curative resection of adrenocortical carcinoma. Journal of the American Medical Association Surgery. 2016;**151**(4):365-373

[8] Fassnacht M, Arlt W, Bancos I, Dralle H, Newell-Price J, Sahdev A, et al. Management of adrenal incidentalomas: European Society of Endocrinology Clinical Practice

Guideline in collaboration with the European Network for the Study of Adrenal Tumors. European Journal of Endocrinology/European Federation of Endocrine Societies. 2016;**175**(2):G1-G34

[9] Zeiger MA, Thompson GB, Duh QY, Hamrahian AH, Angelos P, Elaraj D, et al. American Association of Clinical Endocrinologists and American Association of Endocrine Surgeons Medical Guidelines for the management of adrenal incidentalomas: Executive summary of recommendations. Endocrine Practice: Official Journal of the American College of Endocrinology and the American Association of Clinical Endocrinologists. 2009;**15**(5):450-453

[10] Bharwani N, Rockall AG, Sahdev A, Gueorguiev M, Drake W, Grossman AB, et al. Adrenocortical carcinoma: The range of appearances on CT and MRI. AJR American Journal of Roentgenology. 2011;**196**(6):W706-W714

[11] Schieda N, Al Dandan O, Kielar AZ, Flood TA, McInnes MD, Siegelman ES. Pitfalls of adrenal imaging with chemical shift MRI. Clinical Radiology. 2014;**69**(11):1186-1197

[12] Boland GW, Dwamena BA, Jagtiani Sangwaiya M, Goehler AG, Blake MA, Hahn PF, et al. Characterization of adrenal masses by using FDG PET: Asystematic review and meta-analysis of diagnostic test performance. Radiology. 2011;**259**(1):117-126

[13] Groussin L, Bonardel G, Silvera S, Tissier F, Coste J, Abiven G, et al. 18F-Fluorodeoxyglucose positron emission tomography for the diagnosis of adrenocortical tumors: A prospective study in 77 operated patients. The Journal of Clinical Endocrinology and Metabolism. 2009;**94**(5):1713-1722

[14] Lenders JW, Pacak K, Walther MM, Linehan WM, Mannelli M, Friberg P, et al. Biochemical diagnosis of pheochromocytoma: Which test is best? JAMA: The Journal of the American Medical Association. 2002;**287**(11):1427-1434

[15] Rossi GP, Barisa M, Allolio B, Auchus RJ, Amar L, Cohen D, et al. The Adrenal Vein Sampling International Study (AVIS) for identifying the major subtypes of primary aldosteronism. The Journal of Clinical Endocrinology and Metabolism. 2012;**97**(5):1606-1614

[16] Monticone S, Satoh F, Giacchetti G, Viola A, Morimoto R, Kudo M, et al. Effect of adrenocorticotropic hormone stimulation during adrenal vein sampling in primary aldosteronism. Hypertension (Dallas, Tex: 1979). 2012;**59**(4):840-846

[17] Toniato A, Merante-Boschin I, Opocher G, Pelizzo MR, Schiavi F, Ballotta E. Surgical versus conservative management for subclinical Cushing syndrome in adrenal incidentalomas: A prospective randomized study. Annals of Surgery. 2009;**249**(3):388-391

[18] Donatini G, Caiazzo R, Do Cao C, Aubert S, Zerrweck C, El-Kathib Z, et al. Long-term survival after adrenalectomy for stage I/II adrenocortical carcinoma (ACC): A retrospective comparative cohort study of laparoscopic versus open approach. Annals of Surgical Oncology. 2014;**21**(1):284-291

Chapter 2

Unusual Presentations of Adrenal Masses

Santosh Kumar and Shivanshu Singh

Additional information is available at the end of the chapter

http://dx.doi.org/10.5772/intechopen.69393

Abstract

With the advancement in imaging technology and pathological evaluation, several unusual adrenal gland lesions have been identified over the years. Presently, the literature consists of case reports or small case series without a comprehensive review on these uncommon adrenal pathologies. The current chapter discusses the epidemiology, pathogenesis, pathology, imaging features and management principles of uncommonly reported infectious and neoplastic adrenal masses.

Keywords: tuberculosis, echinococcosis, myelolipoma, oncocytoma, hemangioma

1. Introduction

The diagnosis of unusual adrenal gland masses over the past years has been facilitated by advances in imaging and molecular histopathology. This chapter of unusual adrenal masses as a result of infection, benign or malignant tumors provides the most comprehensive review and recent information on this topic. The epidemiology, clinical presentation, radiologic and pathologic features of atypical adrenal masses as well as their current management will be discussed.

2. Infections presenting as adrenal masses

The adrenal gland can be infected by several pathogens including bacteria, fungi, viruses and parasites. Infections of the adrenal gland are important, but an underreported clinical entity. Such infections can cause either direct adrenal tissue damage during microbial replication and toxin production or indirect damage through alteration of host's immunologic and endocrine response to an infection from a distant site. Disparities in pathogen tropism, adrenal anatomy, and host immune integrity contribute to active disease progression and adrenal dysfunction. Timely diagnosis and management of such adrenal infections significantly improves outcome, thereby highlighting the importance of clinical suspicion in the clinic setting [1].

2.1. Adrenal tuberculosis

In one reported series, the incidence of adrenal involvement was 6% of patients with active tuberculosis [2]. Adrenal glands are infected through a hematogenous route [3]. Clinical manifestations may take years to appear while others may have asymptomatic infections. Tuberculosis must be suspected in patients with a fever along with adrenomegaly [4]. At least 90% of the adrenal gland must be involved with parenchymal destruction before clinical features of adrenal insufficiency appear [5]. Stress and inflammation are thought to be underlying reasons for adrenal enlargement in patients with tuberculosis without microbial seeding of the glands. While few studies have demonstrated elevated basal and stimulated cortisol levels [6], others have shown lower cortisol levels [7].

Imaging studies help in the evaluation of affected adrenal glands (**Figure 1**). Most patients with active or recently acquired disease (within 2 years) have bilateral adrenal enlargement, while the remaining with remote infection or inactive disease have calcifications and/or gland atrophy [5, 8]. In one study, 91% of patients with adrenal tuberculosis who underwent CT had bilaterally enlarged adrenal glands, while 2% had normal sized glands. Among those with adrenal enlargement, mass-like lesions were noted in 49% while enlargement with preserved contours was found in the remaining 51% of patients; more than half of them had peripheral rim enhancement. With longer duration of disease, calcifications and contour preservation were seen more frequently, whereas peripheral rim enhancement and mass-like enlargement seen less significantly on CT images [9]. Adrenal glands may also be enlarged in patients with extra-adrenal tuberculosis. Although not needed in cases of extra-adrenal tuberculosis, an adrenal biopsy may be diagnostic in patients with suspected adrenal tuberculosis without extra-adrenal disease [3, 10].

Treatment includes multiple antituberculosis medications. Studies have demonstrated reduction of gland size after successful treatment of extra-adrenal tuberculosis [11]. In patients with adrenal insufficiency, antituberculosis medications do not effectively restore adrenal function after treatment. Furthermore, steroid replacement therapy may need to be increased as rifampicin induces glucocorticoid metabolism in the liver [12].

2.2. Adrenal histoplasmosis

Adrenal involvement is usually found in patients with disseminated histoplasmosis. The clinical, pathologic and radiologic presentation is similar to that of tuberculosis with diagnosis confirmed by adrenal gland biopsy [13, 14]. In one series, primary adrenal insufficiency was reported in 41% of patients [15]. Populations at risk for adrenal histoplasmosis include immunocompromised, posttransplant and elderly patients [16]. CT usually demonstrates bilaterally enlarged adrenal glands, whereas pathologic examination reveals necrotizing granulomas and caseous necrosis. Differential diagnosis of bilateral adrenomegaly includes lymphoma, metastasis, sarcoidosis, adrenal hemorrhage, and infections like tuberculosis, histoplasmosis,

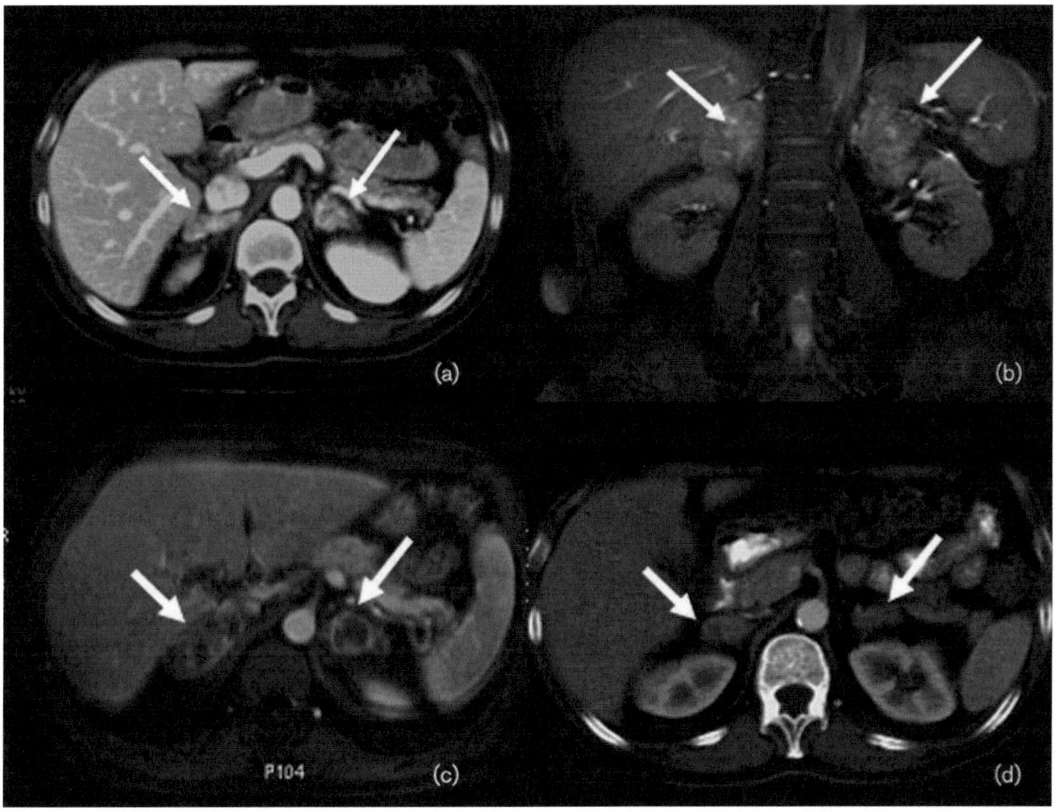

Figure 1. Radiological features of adrenal tuberculosis. (a) Adrenal enlargement with high contrast uptake and rim enhancement demonstrated on CT scan; (b) Adrenal enlargement shown on a coronal FS T1 MRI scan; (c) Adrenal enlargement shown on an axial FS T1 MRI scan; (d) Significant reduction of the volume of the adrenal glands with no pathological contrast uptake on a CT scan after treatment. (Courtesy: Ref. [4].)

cryptococcosis, coccidioidomycosis and blastomycosis. However, central hypodensity and peripheral rim enhancement of the adrenal glands by CT narrows the differential diagnosis to histoplasmosis and tuberculosis only [17]. Recommended antifungal therapy includes amphotericin B followed by itraconazole (for disseminated disease), and glucocorticoid and mineralocorticoid replacement for adrenal insufficiency.

2.3. Adrenal cryptococcosis

Cryptococcal infections most commonly present as pneumonia or meningitis with adrenal glands only usually involved in immunocompromised patients with disseminated cryptococcal infection [18]. However, cases of isolated adrenal gland involvement have been reported [19]. CT can demonstrate enlarged adrenal glands [20], and diagnosis is confirmed by a biopsy that shows budding yeasts with capsules on smear examination with India ink or methenamine silver stain (**Figure 2**). In most cases, cryptococcal antigen titers are elevated and used as a biomarker for disease resolution [21]. Intensive Amphotericin B therapy followed by oral fluconazole consolidation (usually 6-month course) is an effective multidrug treatment regimen

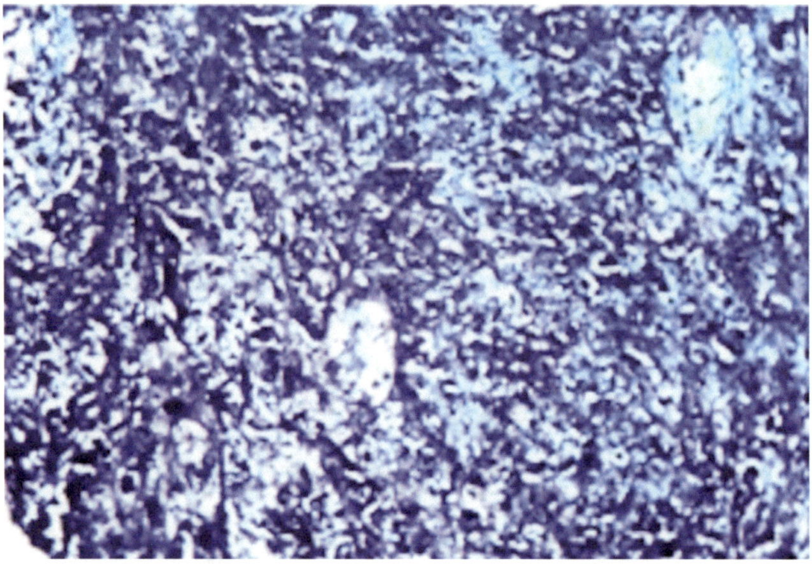

Figure 2. Microscopic examination of cryptococcal infection. Methenamine silver stain shows the yeast, some of which demonstrate budding (40x). (Courtesy: Ref. [22].)

[22, 23]. In contrast to adrenal tuberculosis and histoplasmosis, adrenal insufficiency is often improved with resolution of this infection. Adrenal cryptococcal infection resistant to antifungal therapy may respond to adrenalectomy [24].

3. Parasitic infections of the adrenal glands

Parasitic infections of the adrenal glands are rarely reported, and their prevalence depends on the organism, residence in endemic areas and host immune integrity [1]. The nature of adrenal gland involvement varies significantly depending on the microbe. Case reports have shown adrenal involvement with a wide range of pathogens that includes *Echinococcus, Leishmania, Trypanosoma, Microsporidia* and amebic species.

3.1. Adrenal echinococcosis

Echinococcal infections of the adrenal glands are uncommon, accounting for 6–7% of all cysts [25–27]. Adrenal involvement is usually secondary, and part of generalized echinococcosis [25, 28]. Most cases are discovered incidentally, although some cases present with nonspecific dull aching flank pain [29]. Adrenal hydatids can cause hypertension, known as "the Goldblatt phenomenon", due to irritation of functional tissue of the adrenal gland by the growing cyst [30].

Imaging studies are helpful in characterizing infected adrenal cysts, and ultrasonography (US) is particularly helpful in securing the diagnosis. US of the adrenal cyst can demonstrate location, size and number along with cyst features that include floating membranes, daughter cysts, multiple septa and hydatids. The WHO/IWG-E classification for diagnosis and treatment of echinococcal cysts is based on US imaging characteristics that classify cysts into six subtypes (CL, CE1 to CE5) and three relevant groups: active (CE1 and 2), transitional (CE3) and inactive (CE4 and 5) [31]. On CT, unilocular or multilocular cysts are identified with debris, calcified walls, small daughter cysts and increased tissue density of hydatid membrane, which shows contrast enhancement [32]. CT provides information regarding the cyst number, origin and residual parenchyma of the affected organ, and relationship of the cyst with adjacent structures. Serological tests are marred by low sensitivity and specificity. Latest immunodiagnostic tests detect echinococcal antigens in hydatid fluid fraction. These tests detect *Echinococcus granulosus* antigen 5, *E. granulosus* antigen B (AgB), and EpC1. AgB8/2 antigen has shown maximum diagnostic sensitivity (84–93%) and specificity (98–99%) [33, 34]. Serology is helpful in continued patient monitoring as titers decrease following definitive therapy [35].

Multiple therapeutic options include medical therapy, percutaneous intervention, open and minimally invasive laparoscopic and robotic surgeries. Surgical excision usually results in definitive cure. Medical therapy is usually implemented as an adjunct to surgical excision. Antiparasitic medications as primary treatment is recommended for cases with disseminated hydatidosis, brain or bony echinococcosis or in patients with poor surgical risk [32]. Preoperative oral therapy with albendazole (10–15 mg/kg per day) with or without praziquantel (50 mg/kg) for 4 weeks before surgery may kill scolices, make the cyst inactive, decrease cyst material antigenicity, reduce cyst wall tension and thereby reduce the risk of spillage [26]. In liver echinococcosis, studies have shown a lower risk of recurrence following surgery in cases that had received preoperative albendazole versus those who did not (4 vs. 19%), respectively [36]. Limitations of medical therapy include serious drug-related adverse effects such as leukopenia, hepatotoxicity, allergic reactions and alopecia [37], and limited experience in its use in genitourinary echinococcosis.

Surgical management involves adrenal hydatid cyst excision by laparoscopic or open techniques [29]. It is difficult to determine whether complete excision of adrenal is mandatory as data is limited. In a series of nine cases, adrenalectomy was performed in patients with adrenal cysts with no recurrence at a median follow-up of 16 months (range: 6–64 months) [25]. In another study, transperitoneal laparoscopic aspiration with instillation of scolicidal agent with partial cystectomy for an adrenal hydatid cyst was performed (**Figure 3**). The cyst densely adhered to the renal vessels and complete excision involved risk of nephrectomy. Betadine soaked gauze pieces were packed around the cyst. The cyst was aspirated followed by instillation of scolicidal agent that was maintained for 10 min. A 10-mm trocar was introduced into the cyst, and its contents, including the germinal layer, were suctioned and followed by partial cyst wall excision. No recurrence was noted at 6-months follow-up. The authors concluded that total adrenal gland excision may be needed only in cases with complete gland destruction [38]. Complete evacuation of cyst contents and prevention of viable scolices spillage intraperitoneally remains a key principle in the management of adrenal hydatid cysts.

3.2. Other adrenal infections presenting as cysts/masses

Visceral leishmaniasis can present with cystic adrenal disease in both immunocompetent and immunocompromised individuals [39, 40]. Rarely, amebic species have been found in cystic lesions of the adrenal gland [1]. *Trypanosoma cruzi*, the causative agent of Chagas disease, has

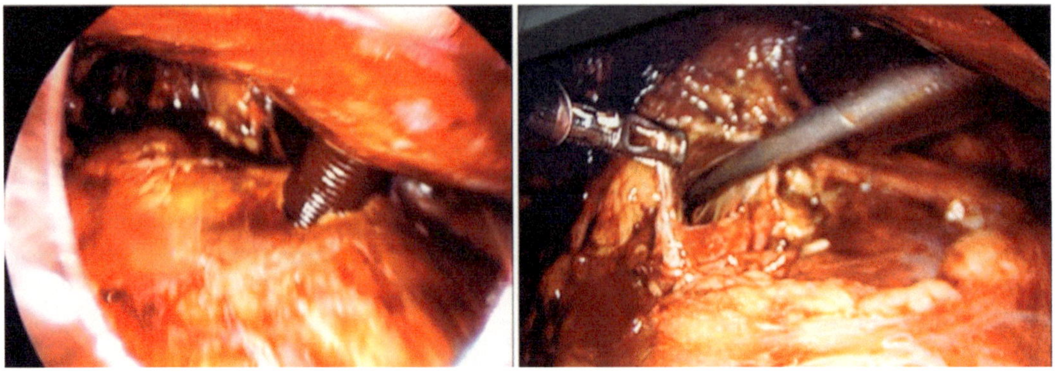

Figure 3. Laparoscopic management of adrenal hydatid cysts. Intraoperative photograph showing cyst aspiration by directly inserting a trocar into the cyst and laparoscopic cyst dissection after aspiration. (Courtesy: Ref. [38].)

been found in infected adrenal glands, which may serve as a reservoir. Investigators have found a correlation between central vein infection of the adrenal gland and development of chagasic myocarditis [41]. African trypanosomiasis has been found to be associated with polyendocrinopathies including hypothyroidism, hypogonadism and adrenal insufficiency resulting from either primary gland or secondary (central) involvement. In a series of 137 patients, adrenal and thyroid function recovered with medical treatment, but hypogonadism tended to persist for years [42]. Two drugs, benznidazole, and nifurtimox are available for treatment of *T. cruzi* infection. However, both benznidazole and nifurtimox are limited in their capacity to provide a parasitologic cure, especially in chronically infected patients [43]. Adrenal involvement from disseminated microsporidia in immunocompromised patients induces large necrotic lesions with histiocytic and fibrotic reactions within the gland substrate [44].

HIV infection affects the adrenal gland in several ways. Apart from direct infection, opportunistic infections and antiretroviral medications also have a significant effect on adrenal glands that can lead to adrenal insufficiency. Cases with HIV infection can harbor adrenal tumors like Kaposi's sarcoma secondary to co-infection with oncogenic human herpesvirus type 8 (HHV8), and non-Hodgkin's lymphoma (high-grade malignant B phenotype) secondary to Epstein-Barr virus (EBV) infection [45, 46].

4. Adrenal tumors

This section describes uncommon benign and malignant adrenal tumors and current concepts in their management.

4.1. Adrenal leiomyoma

Leiomyoma of the adrenal glands is extremely rare tumors with less than 20 cases reported in the literature [47]. Although benign tumors, they may mimic malignant adrenal tumors on radiologic imaging. Age at presentation in patients ranges from 2 to 72 years with 61% usually occurring in women. Tumor size varies from 3 to 11 cm in diameter [48]. Usually asymptomatic and nonfunctional, such tumors present as adrenal incidentalomas and occasionally as calcified masses [49]. Some patients may present with vague, nonspecific flank or upper abdominal pain. Many cases of adrenal leiomyomas have been reported to occur in patients with acquired immune deficiency syndrome (AIDS), or latent Epstein-Barr infection [48, 50]. Associated smooth-muscle tumors and Kaposi's sarcoma may arise from a common stem cell under the influence of some unknown factor produced during HIV infection [51]. Grossly, cut sections often demonstrate a whorled appearance. Light microscopy shows spindle-shaped cells arranged in fascicles and whorls (**Figure 4**) [47]. Immunohistochemistry helps in establishing a diagnosis as the tumor cells show diffuse and strong positivity for smooth muscle actin [52]. Prognosis is good following complete surgical resection. With the advent of minimally invasive surgery, laparoscopic resection is feasible with good perioperative outcomes [49]. Large tumors, however, do pose challenges for adjacent vital organ preservation during surgical resection.

4.2. Inflammatory myofibroblastic tumor (IMT)

Inflammatory myofibroblastic tumor (IMT) was first described in 1939. Previously known as plasma cell granuloma or inflammatory pseudotumor, the term "inflammatory myofibroblastic tumor" was introduced in 1986 [53–55]. Although found in the adrenal glands, the most common site of IMT is the lung followed by the orbit [55].

Cytogenetic and molecular advancements have confirmed the neoplastic nature of IMT and their recurrence potential [56, 57]. They exhibit cytogenetic clonality, the involvement of chromosomal region 2p23, occasional aggressive local behavior, and metastasis described in most locations, in both sexes and at all ages [58, 59]. Mean tumor size at the time of presentation ranges from 5 to 10 cm. IMT usually present as an adrenal incidentaloma, although 10–20% of

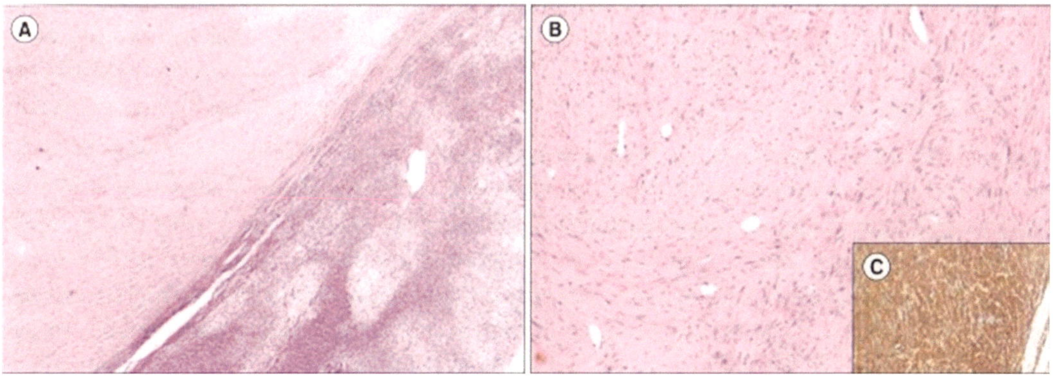

Figure 4. Histopathologic images of adrenal leiomyoma. (A) Normal adrenal gland seen at the periphery with encapsulated tumor arranged in long and short fascicles (H&E, ×40). (B) Higher magnification showing fascicles of benign spindle-shaped cells with minimal nuclear atypia (H&E, × 200). (C) Neoplastic cells showing strong positivity with smooth muscle actin (immunoperoxidase, ×200). (Courtesy: Ref. [49].)

patients have a fever, weight loss or flank pain [60]. These lesions do not demonstrate specific imaging features [60]. Enhanced CT may show heterogeneity or homogeneity of a hypo-, iso- or hyperdense adrenal mass [61].

Grossly, IMT appears firm, fleshy or gelatinous with a white or tan cut surface. Few may also demonstrate calcification, hemorrhage, and necrosis [59]. Histopathology reveals plump fibroblast or myofibroblast proliferation along with prominent infiltrate of chronic inflammatory cells, especially plasma cells. The presence of these plasma cells helps distinguish these adrenal tumors from fibromatosis and fasciitis. The epithelioid variant of IMT is rare with an aggressive clinical course [62]. Histologic markers of aggressive behavior include the presence of ganglion-like cells, cellular atypia, aneuploidy, and p53 overexpression [63]. On immunohistochemistry, these adrenal tumors usually express actin with occasional positivity for desmin and keratin. Thirty to 40% of tumors have ALK protein overexpression as a result of ALK gene rearrangement. Clinical correlation has shown that most patients with tumor metastasis were negative for ALK overexpression [64].

Complete surgical resection is essential since malignancy cannot be excluded preoperatively. Ten to 25% of patients have been reported to have a local recurrence following complete surgical excision. These tumors are considered to be low-grade sarcomas with less than 5% incidence of metastasis. Nevertheless, their biological behavior cannot be predicted based on their morphologic appearance [60].

4.3. Primitive neuroectodermal tumors (PNETs)

Primitive neuroectodermal tumors (PNETs) are associated with a family of small round cell tumors. Initially described a century ago by Arthur Stout in a 42-year male with an ulnar nerve tumor, it was not until 1973 when Hart and Earle coined the term "primitive neuroectodermal tumor" for such unspecialized small round cell tumors [65, 66]. PNETs are classified as central (arising from the central nervous system) and peripheral [67]. Peripheral PNETs that arise from the adrenal glands are extremely rare with less than two-dozen cases reported in the literature. They usually present as a large (>10 cm), nonfunctioning adrenal mass often associated with abdominal pain and metastasis. These solid and/or cystic lesions can rapidly grow and are difficult to differentiate from adrenocortical carcinoma (ACC) radiologically [67, 68]. CT can show irregular bordered, diffusively growing, and unevenly enhancing adrenal masses [67].

Both PNETs and Ewing's sarcoma share a unique translocation "t(11;22)(q24q12): fusion gene designated EWS/FLI-1" [69]. FLI-1 is a member of ETS family of transcription factors [69]. Microscopic examination along with immunohistochemistry helps establish the diagnosis. On light microscopy, classic features include small round cell tumors arranged in nests/rosettes (**Figure 5**). These cells have little endoplasm with dark stained nucleus high in nucleoplasm [67]. Among all the markers, Mic-2 (CD-99) is the most sensitive and specific marker (nearly 100%), which is a cell surface glycoprotein coded by genes on X and Y-chromosomes [70]. Other common markers of neural differentiation include neuron-specific enolase (NSE), S-100 protein, neurofilaments, synaptophysin (Syn), chromogranin A (CgA) and vimentin. The most reliable findings for pathologic diagnosis of PNETs are the existence of rosettes, and two or more positive results of the aforementioned neural markers [67, 71–73].

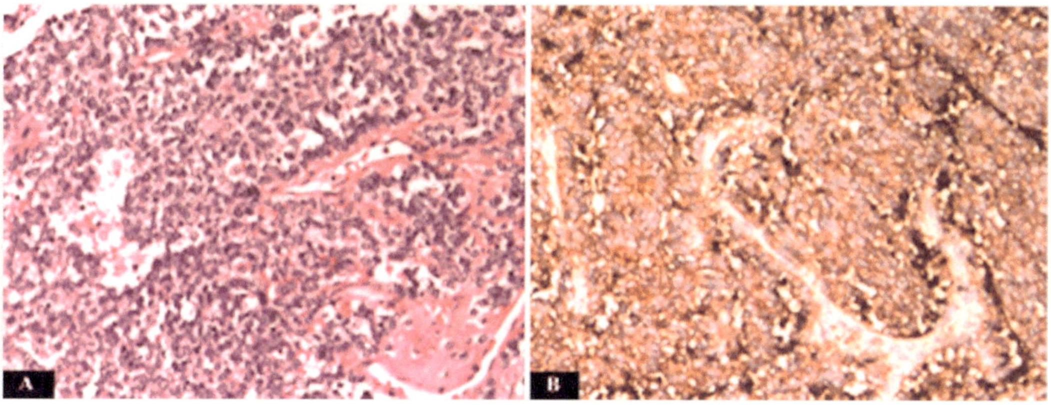

Figure 5. Microscopic picture of adrenal primitive neuroectodermal tumor. (A) Hematoxylin and eosin stains for adrenal primitive neuroectodermal tumor (20×). (B) CD99 Immunohistochemical stains for adrenal primitive neuroectodermal tumor (20×). (Courtesy: Ref. [67].)

Since adrenal PNETs are an uncommon clinical entity, an effective treatment protocol is not yet established. Surgical excision remains the mainstay for local disease control. Adrenalectomy is usually followed by adjuvant radiochemotherapy [74]. A recommended regimen is the alternating use of CAV (cyclophosphamide: CTX; adriamycin: ADM; and vincristine: VCR), and IE (ifosfamide: IFO; and etoposide: ETO) protocols as PNET rapidly develop resistance to a particular regimen [75]. In general, 5-year survival of patients with PNETs is 58–61% with a median survival of 120 months. Local or distant metastasis at the time of diagnosis is associated with poor outcome [70].

4.4. Adrenal oncocytoma

Adrenal oncocytomas are rare tumors. Although considered benign and nonfunctional, these adrenal masses are malignant in 20% and hormonally active in 10–20% of patients [76]. Adrenal oncocytomas have been described in a wide age group (27–72 years) and usually discovered as incidentalomas [77]. Women are more commonly affected [78] with a predominance of the left adrenal gland (3.5:1) [79].

Such adrenal tumors are classified as either benign, borderline malignant potential or malignant using the Lin-Weiss-Bisceglia system that includes the major criteria of high mitotic rate > 5 per 50 HPF, atypical mitoses, venous invasion; and minor criteria that include large size and weight, necrosis, capsular invasion, sinusoidal invasion [80]. The presence of one major criterion indicates malignancy, and one to four minor criteria indicates uncertain malignant potential. The absence of all major and minor criteria indicates a benign adrenal tumor.

Microscopically, tumor cells have abundant eosinophilic granular cytoplasm due to the accumulation of mitochondria with a central pyknotic nucleus [81]. They may be arranged in trabecular, tubular, papillary or solid patterns. The classic central stellate scar of renal oncocytoma may not be seen. Immunophenotyping, in general, reveals diffuse positivity for vimentin, melan-A, synaptophysin and alpha-inhibin [82].

Due to its large size and lack of characteristic preoperative imaging features for benignity, surgical resection remains the principal management for adrenal oncocytomas [79]. Surgical excision is a challenging task in giant adrenal oncocytomas (**Figure 6**). Although not infiltrating, the large size of these tumors can alter the orientation and position of adjacent viscera and major blood vessels. *En bloc* mobilization of spleen, stomach, and pancreas helps provide optimum exposure for large left-sided adrenal oncocytomas [83].

4.5. Adrenal myelolipoma

First described in 1905, adrenal myelolipoma is a rare adrenal tumor with a prevalence of <1% in autopsy series [84]. These adrenal tumors have an overall incidence of 0.05–0.2%, and account for about 2.5–5% of all adrenal incidentalomas. Both women and men are equally affected, and they are usually unilateral and rarely arise from extra-adrenal sites such as the retroperitoneum, thorax, and pelvis [85]. Symptomatic patients may present with abdominal pain or uncommonly with massive hemorrhage and shock, or with fever and abscess [85]. Tumor size varies widely from a few centimeters to >30 cm [84]. Although the tumor is metabolically inactive, there is a 10% incidence of associated endocrine disorders such as Cushing's and Conn's syndromes, congenital adrenal hyperplasia and diabetes [86].

These adrenal lesions are also rarely associated with thalassemia and sickle cell anemia [87, 88]. For reasons not yet understood, myelolipomas in patients with thalassemia are usually giant and bilateral. Such association might be due to excess erythropoietin production [89]. Various mechanisms have been proposed regarding its pathogenesis. These tumors are

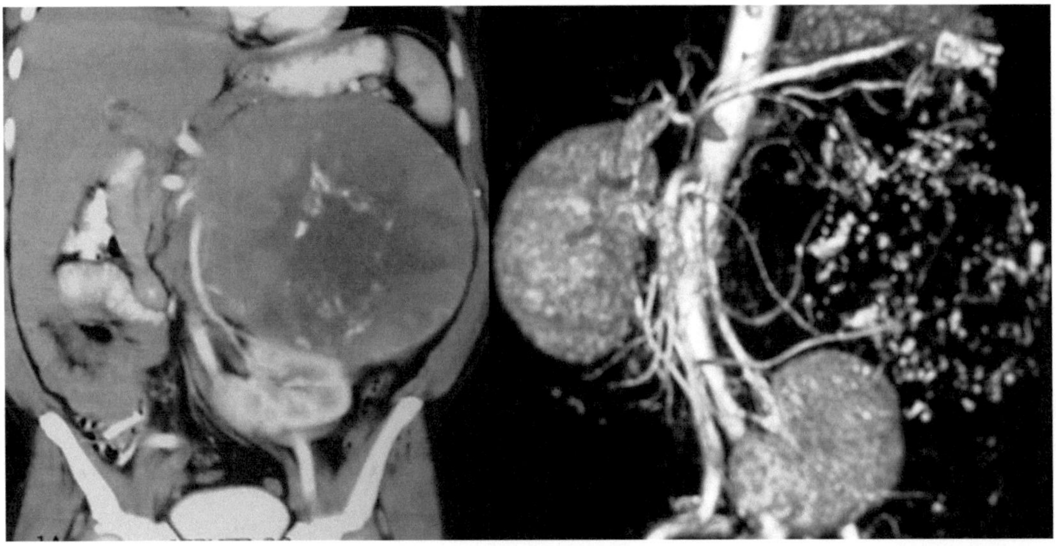

Figure 6. CT in preoperative planning in case of giant adrenal oncocytoma. Coronal section of contrast enhanced CT demonstrating a giant left adrenal oncocytoma with left kidney lying in transverse plane at iliac crest. The left renal vessels are stretched over the inferolateral aspect of the adrenal mass. CT-angiography shows multiple feeding vessels to the tumor.

believed to arise from metaplasia of reticuloendothelial cells of blood capillaries within the adrenal glands in response to inflammation, necrosis, infection, or stress [84]. Studies have shown nonrandom X-chromosome inactivation in hematopoietic lineage and fat cells, and balanced translocations between 3q25 and 21p11 suggestive of clonal origin [90, 91]. Tumor tissue consists of an admixture of mature adipose tissue, normal trilineage hematopoietic elements, and an overabundance of megakaryocytes. Unlike normal bone marrow, their cellularity varies widely that does not decrease with advanced age. These lesions do not contribute to hematopoietic cells in circulation due to stromal irregularities and lack of capillary venous sinuses [90]. In most cases, this diagnosis can be made accurately on cross-sectional imaging. CT demonstrates a well-circumscribed lesion with a variable amount of mature adipose tissue with low attenuation value (around-30 Hounsfield units) with higher density myeloid component that enhances on contrast administration (**Figure 7**). Nearly one-fourth of cases have calcifications while many have hemorrhagic areas [85]. Rare differential diagnoses include adrenal lipomas, teratomas, liposarcomas, metastasis and upper polar renal angiomyolipoma. Percutaneous biopsy may be helpful when the diagnosis is in doubt [92].

Surgical resection is the mainstay of definitive treatment; however, it is reserved for symptomatic or large adrenal myelolipomas. Small and asymptomatic adrenal lesions can be followed as they remain stable or even decrease in size over long periods of time [92]. In one study, the calculated doubling time of adrenal myelolipomas ranged from 4.6 to 95.1 months (mean 31.9 months) that confirmed the relatively slow growing nature of these tumors [93]. Spontaneous rupture of these lesions is a rare event and usually, occurs in lesions > 10 cm [94].

4.6. Adrenal schwannoma

Schwannomas are benign, well-encapsulated tumors arising from the nerve sheaths of cranial and peripheral nerves [95]. Initially described by Verocay and later subclassified by Antonini

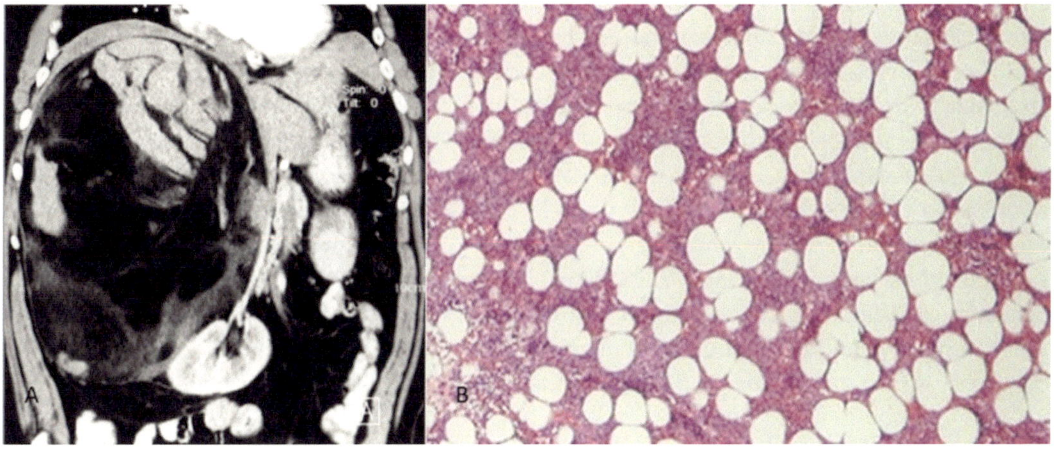

Figure 7. Adrenal myelolipoma. (A) Enhanced CT abdomen showing a 35 × 19 cm right suprarenal mass with areas of macroscopic fat densities (−19 HU) along with focal areas of enhancement. (B) Histopathology showing mature adipocytes admixed with hematopoietic cells suggestive of myelolipoma.

in 1920, they account for 1–5% of all retroperitoneal tumors [96, 97]. Adrenal schwannomas are very rare and restricted to a few case reports. In the adrenal glands, these tumors are believed to arise from Schwann cells surrounding the nerves innervating the adrenal medulla [98]. They may present either as incidentalomas or with abdominal pain. Nonfunctional by nature, positive biochemical evaluation of an adrenal incidentaloma excludes the diagnosis of a schwannoma [96]. CT scan reveals a well-circumscribed, homogeneous, round-oval mass with calcification or cystic degeneration [99]. MRI findings are nonspecific and demonstrate solid tumors with low signal intensity on T1WI and heterogeneously high intensity on T2WI [100]. 18FDG–PET is helpful in differentiating benign from malignant adrenal masses based on standardized uptake value (SUV) [101].

Treatment of choice for adrenal schwannomas is complete surgical excision. Histologic examination reveals characteristic Antoni α and Antoni β areas seen under the microscope, and also nuclear free zones known as Verocay bodies that confirm the diagnosis of Schwannoma. The role of immunohistochemical markers including S-100 and vimentin cannot be overlooked as they are used for final confirmation in addition to the typical pattern described above [97, 98]. They also stain positive for laminin and collagen IV, and negative for desmin, keratin, actin, CD34 and CD117 [97]. A positive stain for calretinin is helpful in differentiating Schwannoma from neurofibroma [102]. Although prognosis is usually good following complete surgical resection, the possibility of local recurrence and malignant formation in benign Schwannomas does remain [103].

4.7. Adrenal ganglioneuroma

Adrenal ganglioneuromas are extremely rare benign neuroectodermal tumors composed of ganglion and Schwann cells [104]. These tumors are predominantly found in younger populations with 50% of patients between 10 and 29 years of age [104]. Although benign, isolated case reports of ganglioneuroma undergoing malignant transformation, cases of peripheral nerve sheath tumors arising within ganglioneuromas, and composite tumors of ganglioneuroma with pheochromocytoma have been reported in the literature [104, 105]. Most ganglioneuromas are asymptomatic, however, some patients with these tumors may present with diarrhea as they have been reported to secrete vasoactive intestinal polypeptide (VIP) [104, 105]. These tumors can grow to large size with blood vessel encasement without compromising the vascular lumen [105]. The biologic and radiologic features that should raise the suspicion of ganglioneuroma include: no adrenal hormone hyperactivity; presence of punctuate calcifications, no vascular involvement, nonenhanced CT attenuation of <40 Hounsfield units (HU); a homogeneous, hypointense mass on T1-weighted MRI; heterogeneous, hyperintense adrenal mass on T2-weighted MRI; and poor, delayed enhancement on dynamic MRI [106]. Histopathology reveals mature ganglion cells and Schwann cells among a fibrous stroma. Complete surgical resection of these adrenal masses is the treatment of choice. Although adrenal ganglioneuromas may encase major vessels at the time of surgery, organ preservation is feasible, as these tumors do not infiltrate them [107].

4.8. Adrenal lipoma

Adrenal lipomas are rare adrenal masses with the majority predominantly occurring in men with a range from 35 to 78 years of age [108]. These lesions account for 0.7% of all lipomatous adrenal tumors [109]. These tumors are more common on the right side with a size ranging from 1 to 20 cm [110]. Although usually asymptomatic, patients with larger tumors may experience abdominal pain whereas few patients may present with an acute abdomen due to retroperitoneal bleeding [111], and a smaller minority with hypertension [112]. These adrenal masses are thought to arise from metaplasia of either stromal or adrenal cortical cells [113]. CT demonstrates a well-defined adrenal lesion with fat densities without enhancing hematopoietic tissue as seen in myelolipomas. Microscopic examination reveals well-demarcated lesions composed of mature adipose lobules with occasional focal areas of calcification due to degenerative changes [113]. Surgical excision is curative. Although the laparoscopic approach is preferred, it is difficult to perform in giant adrenal lipomas and those complicated by rupture, bleeding or sarcomatous changes [114].

4.9. Cystic pheochromocytoma

Cystic pheochromocytomas are rare adrenal masses thought to arise as a result of bleeding, necrosis, and liquefaction within solid pheochromocytomas. Patients with such adrenal lesions are more likely to be asymptomatic with occasional nonspecific abdominal symptoms and may have a normal biochemical profile when compared to solid tumors [115, 116]. CT often reveals a thick walled cystic lesion with presence or absence of septa within the adrenal mass, and persistent wall enhancement after contrast administration [115]. Surgical excision is the most definitive treatment of pheochromocytomas regardless of whether the tumor is cystic or not [117]. It is essential to consider this diagnosis in the differential as normotensive patients with unsuspected cystic pheochromocytoma have been reported to have intraoperative hypertensive crises during surgical excision [118].

4.10. Adrenal plasmacytoma (extramedullary plasmacytoma)

Extramedullary plasmacytoma (EMP) is defined as an extraosseous proliferation of neoplastic plasma cells. These adrenal tumors are cytogenetically identical to plasma cell myeloma but occur as isolated lesions [119]. Solitary EMP of the adrenal glands is extremely rare with fewer than a dozen cases reported in the literature. These adrenal masses usually occur in men than women (3:1) within the age range of 50–60 years [120]. The most common site of solitary EMP is the head and neck region followed by the gastrointestinal tract [121]. Although plasma cell proliferation caused by trauma might ultimately lead to clonal cell infiltration, pathogenesis of such tumors remains unclear [122]. Preoperative imaging of these lesions has heterogeneous hyperintensity on T2-weighted images.

Definitive diagnosis of adrenal plasmacytoma is based on the pathologic confirmation of a solitary plasma cell tumor, with or without a monoclonal gammopathy, and the absence of plasma cell myeloma on bone marrow biopsy [119]. Pathologic examination reveals dense and diffuse infiltrate of atypical plasma cells with very few admixed lymphocytes. Immunohistochemistry shows monoclonal immunoglobulin light chain expression. The diagnosis of solitary EMP can be confirmed after excluding systemic disease by serum and urine protein electrophoresis, immunoelectrophoresis, skeletal imaging survey, and bone marrow biopsy. Staging bone marrow biopsy is essential to exclude plasma cell myeloma [121].

A standard treatment protocol has not been established for adrenal EMP. In cases with solitary lesions, complete surgical resection with or without radiotherapy has been reported with good outcomes in term of disease-free status [122–124]. In one report, bilateral adrenal EMP was treated by chemotherapy and autologous hematopoietic stem cell transplantation with no recurrence at 47 months follow-up [125].

4.11. Non-Hodgkin lymphoma (NHL) of adrenal glands

Primary adrenal lymphoma is defined as a malignant neoplastic proliferation of lymphoid cells exclusively within the adrenal tissue. The adrenal glands are involved in up to 24% of patients with disseminated lymphoma [126]. Isolated primary adrenal lymphoma is rare, and constitutes 3% of extranodal lymphoma [127]. Bilateral adrenal involvement is reported in 70% of patients [128]. Most cases are found in the elderly with a male to female ratio of 2:1. The most common subtype found in the adrenal glands is diffuse large B-cell lymphoma [126]. Multi-agent chemotherapy that includes cyclophosphamide, hydroxyl-doxorubicin (adriamycin), vincristine (oncovin), and prednisolone (CHOP) along with rituximab for CD20 positive cases represents the cornerstone of management [129]. When an isolated adrenal mass, diagnosis is usually made following adrenalectomy. However, adjuvant chemotherapy is given to prevent disease recurrence [126]. Prognostic factors that include age, elevated serum lactate dehydrogenase, adrenal insufficiency and tumor size may have a significant impact on treatment outcome and survival. Prognosis for patients has slightly improved with recent chemotherapeutic agents. Although a median survival of nearly 3 months was previously reported [130], most recent data in the literature suggests disease free status of 12 months [126].

4.12. Adrenal hemangioma

Adrenal hemangiomas are rare benign tumors. These lesions arise from the endothelial cell lining of blood vessels. Adrenal hemangiomas are believed to be congenital in origin with enlargement of >10 cm at the time of presentation as a result of vascular ectasia [131]. They are usually detected in 6 to 7th decade of life. Women are twice more commonly affected than men, and most cases occur unilaterally [132]. Patients are usually asymptomatic, although spontaneous life-threatening hemorrhage from adrenal hemangiomas has been reported [133]. Cases of bilateral adrenal hemangioma can also occur [134]. CT reveals heterogeneous, hypodense lesions with a high-density rim of tissue at the periphery [131]. Contrast-enhanced CT scans show peripheral spotty contrast with centripetal enhancement; this enhancement pattern is pathognomonic for hemangiomas. Certain patterns of calcification have also been reported, and include either speckled calcifications throughout the lesion or centrally located calcifications with an irregular, stellate branching pattern [135]. MRI reveals marked hyperintensity on T2-weighted images and focal hyperintensity on T1-weighted images with focal areas of hemorrhage [136]. Pathologic examination reveals multiple dilated vascular channels lined by single layer of endothelium with areas of hemorrhage, necrosis, and calcification [131]. Tumor size and symptoms help determine the need for surgical intervention in patients where characteristic imaging features make the diagnosis of adrenal hemangioma; lesions < 3.5 cm can be safely observed by serial imaging studies [137]. Surgical excision is recommended for larger lesions, symptomatic patients or in those patients where imaging features are atypical.

5. Surgical excision of giant adrenal tumors

Since the adrenal glands are situated in the retroperitoneum, various vital organs lie in close vicinity. Giant benign adrenal tumors pose challenges for safe surgical resection with preservation of vital organs such as kidneys, spleen, mesenteric and great vessels. One such technique is *en bloc* mobilization of the pancreas and spleen for large left adrenal masses derived from multi-visceral transplantation techniques [83]. Prompt recognition and management of vascular injury can prevent catastrophe. In a case report of a giant left adrenocortical carcinoma where the superior mesenteric artery (SMA) was injured due to anatomical distortion, prompt recognition followed by end-to-end anastomosis salvaged the SMA [138]. At times, major vascular resection with the placement of a prosthesis may be required. Certain operative principles for giant adrenal tumors include a thorough knowledge of retroperitoneal anatomy, careful and meticulous dissection, enhanced CT with 3D reconstructions for delineating relationship of the adrenal tumor to the surrounding structures, a low threshold for conversion to open procedure, use of specialized vessel sealing devices that can secure small parasitic vessels with minimal collateral thermal damage; and adherence to oncologic goals for complete surgical excision to minimize disease recurrence.

6. Conclusion

Knowledge of unusual adrenal masses is essential for those clinicians involved in the management of adrenal disorders. This chapter has provided a comprehensive review of the pathogenesis, clinical presentation, and management of uncommon adrenal masses.

Acknowledgements

Authors confirm the copyright permission for use of pictures throughout the chapter.

Author details

Santosh Kumar* and Shivanshu Singh

*Address all correspondence to: santoshsp1967jaimatadi@yahoo.co.in

Department of Urology, Advanced Urology Center, Postgraduate Institute of Medical Education and Research, Chandigarh, India

References

[1] Paolo WF Jr, Nosanchuk JD. Adrenal infections. International Journal of Infectious Diseases. 2006;**10**:343–353

[2] Lam KY, Lo CY. A critical examination of adrenal tuberculosis and a 28-year autopsy experience of active tuberculosis. Clinical Endocrinology. 2001;**54**:633–639

[3] Upadhyay J, Sudhindra P, Abraham G, Trivedi N. Tuberculosis of the adrenal gland: A case report and review of the literature of infections of the adrenal gland. International Journal of Endocrinology. 2014;**2014**:876037

[4] Borgo CD, Urigo C, Marocco R, Belvisi V, Pisani L, Citton R. et al. Diagnostic and therapeutic approach in a rare case of primary bilateral adrenal tuberculosis. Journal of Medical Microbiology.2010:**59**:1527–1529

[5] Kelestimur F. The endocrinology of adrenal tuberculosis: the effects of tuberculosis on the hypothalamo-pituitary-adrenal axis and adrenocortical function. Journal of Endocrinological Investigation. 2004;**27**:380–386

[6] Keleştimur F, Göktaş Z, GülmezI, Ünlühizarci K, Bayram F, Özesmi M. et al. Low dose (1 μg) adrenocorticotropin stimulation test in the evaluation of hypothalamo-pituitary-adrenal axis in patients with active pulmonary tuberculosis. Journal of Endocrinological Investigation. 2000:**23**:235–239

[7] Laway BA, Khan I, Shah BA, Choh NA, Bhat MA, Shah ZA. Pattern of adrenal morphology and function in pulmonary tuberculosis: Response to treatment with antitubercular therapy. Clinical Endocrinology. 2013;**79**:321–325

[8] McMurry JF, Long D, McClure R, Kotchen TA. Addison's disease with adrenal enlargement on computed tomographic scanning: Report of two cases of tuberculosis and review of the literature. The American journal of medicine. 1984;**77**:365–368

[9] Guo YK, Yang ZG, Li Y, Ma ES, Deng YP, Min PQ. et al. Addison's disease due to adrenal tuberculosis: contrast-enhanced CT features and clinical duration correlation. European Journal of Radiology. 2007;**62**:126–131

[10] Kelestimur F, Unlu Y, Ozesmi M, Tolu I. A hormonal and radiological evaluation of adrenal gland in patients with acute or chronic pulmonary tuberculosis. Clinical Endocrinology. 1994:**41**:53–56

[11] Gülmez I, Kelestimur F, Durak AC, Özesmi M. Changes in the size of adrenal glands in acute pulmonary tuberculosis with therapy. Endocrine Journal. 1996;**43**:573–576

[12] Bhatia E, Jain SK, Gupta RK, Pandey R. Tuberculous Addison's disease: Lack of normalization of adrenocortical function after anti-tuberculous chemotherapy. Clinical Endocrinology. 1998;**48**:355–359

[13] Goodwin JR RA, Shapiro JL, Thurman GH, Thurman SS, Des Prez RM. Disseminated histoplasmosis: Clinical and pathologic correlations. Medicine. 1 Jan 1980;**59**(1):1–33

[14] Mukherjee JJ, Villa ML, Tan L, Lee KO. Image in endocrinology: Bilateral adrenal masses due to histoplasmosis. The Journal of Clinical Endocrinology and Metabolism. 2005: **90**:6725–6726

[15] Koene RJ, Catanese J, Sarosi GA. Adrenal hypofunction from histoplasmosis: A literature review from 1971 to 2012. Infection. 2013;**41**:757–759

[16] Kauffman CA. Fungal infections in older adults. Clinical Infectious Diseases. 2001;33: 550–555

[17] Vyas S, Kalra N, Das PJ, Lal A, Radhika S, Bhansali A. Adrenal histoplasmosis: An unusual cause of adrenomegaly. Indian Journal of Nephrology. 2011;**21**:283–285

[18] Subramanian S, Mathai D. Clinical manifestations and management of cryptococcal infection. Journal of Postgraduate Medicine. 2005;**51**:S21-S26

[19] Cocker R, McNair SA, Kahn L, Kwon S, Ding X, Zeltsman V. et al. Isolated adrenal cryptococcosis, diagnosed by fine-needle aspiration biopsy: A case report. Diagnostic Cytopathology. 2014;**42**:899–901. DOI: 10.1002/dc.23079

[20] Walker BF, Gunthel CJ, Bryan JA, Watts NB, Clark RV. Disseminated cryptococcosis in an apparently normal host presenting as primary adrenal insufficiency: Diagnosis by fine needle aspiration. American Journal of Medicine. 1989;**86**:715–717

[21] Hung ZS, Lai YH, Hsu YH, Wang CH, FangTC, Hsu BG. Disseminated cryptococcosis causes adrenal insufficiency in an immunocompetent individual. Internal Medicine. 2010;**49**:1023–1026

[22] Ranjan P, Jana M, Krishnan S, Nath D, Sood R. Disseminated cryptococcosis with adrenal and lung involvement in an immunocompetent patient. Journal of Clinical and Diagnostic Research. 2015;**9**:OD04-OD05. DOI: 10.7860/JCDR/2015/11499.5752

[23] Huston SM, Mody CH. Cryptococcosis: An emerging respiratory mycosis. Clinics in Chest Medicine. 2009;**30**:253–264

[24] Takeshita A, Nakazawa H, Akiyama H, Takeuchi K, Kawai R, Oohashi K. et al. Disseminated cryptococcosis presenting with adrenal insufficiency and meningitis: Resistant to prolonged antifungal therapy but responding to bilateral adrenalectomy. Internal Medicine. 1992;**31**:1401–1405

[25] Akcay MN, Akcay G, Balik AA, Boyuk A. Hydatid cysts of the adrenal gland: Review of nine patients. World Journal of Surgery. 2004;**28**:97–99. DOI: 10.4111/kju.2014.55.7.493

[26] Goel MC, Agarwal MR, Misra A. Percutaneous drainage of renal hydatid cyst: Early results and follow-up. British Journal of Urology. 1995;**75**:724–728

[27] Foster DG. Adrenal cysts: Review of literature and report of case. Archives of Surgery. 1966;**92**:131–143

[28] Schoretsanitis G, de Bree E, Melissas J, Tsiftsis D. Primary hydatid cyst of the adrenal gland. Scandinavian Journal of Urology. 1998;**32**:51–53

[29] Kumar S, Singh S. Genitourinary hydatid disease. In: Rodriguez-Morales AJ, editor. Current Topics in Echinococcosis. InTech. 2015. DOI: 10.5772/60904

[30] Yeniyol CO, Minareci S, Ayder AR. Primary cyst hydatid of adrenal: A case report. International Urology and Nephrology. 2000;**32**:227–229

[31] Rexiati M, Mutalifu A, Azhati B, Wang W, Yang H, Sheyhedin I. et al. Diagnosis and surgical treatment of renal hydatid disease: A retrospective analysis of 30 cases. PLoS ONE. 2014;**9**:e96602. DOI: 10.1371/journal.pone.0096602

[32] Kumar S, Pandya S, Agarwal S, Lal A. Laparoscopic management of genitourinary hydatid cyst disease. Journal of Endourology. 2008;**22**:1709–1713

[33] Rott MB, Fernandez V, Farias S, Ceni J, Ferreira HB, Haag KL, et al. Comparative analysis of two different subunits of antigen B from *Echinococcus granulosus*: Gene sequences, expression in *Escherichia coli* and serological evaluation. Acta Tropica. 2000;**75**:331–340

[34] Virginio VG, Hernandez A, Rott MB, Monteiro KM, Zandonai AF, Nieto A, et al. A set of recombinant antigens from *Echinococcus granulosus* with potential for use in the immunodiagnosis of human cystic hydatid disease. Clinical & Experimental Immunology. 2003;**132**(2):309–315

[35] Feki W, Ghozzi S, Khiari R, Ghorbel J, Elarbi H, Khouni H, et al. Multiple unusual locations of hydatid cysts including bladder, psoas muscle and liver. Parasitology International. 2008;**57**:83–86

[36] Arif SH, Shams Ul B, Wani NA, Zargar SA, Wani MA, Tabassum R, et al. Albendazole as an adjuvant to the standard surgical management of hydatid cyst liver. International Journal of Surgery. 2008;**6**:448–451

[37] Von Sinner WN, Hellstorm M, Kavegi I, Norlen BJ. Hydatid disease of urinary tract. Journal of Urology. 1993;**149**:577–580

[38] Kumar S, Nanjappa B, Gowda KK. Laparoscopic management of a hydatid cyst of the adrenal gland. Korean Journal of Urology. 2014;**55**:493–495

[39] Mondain-Miton V, Toussaint-Gari M, Hofman P, Marty P, Carles M, De Salvador F, et al. Atypical leishmaniasis in a patient infected with human immunodeficiency virus. Clinical Infectious Diseases. 1995;**21**:663–665

[40] Brenner DS, Jacobs SC, Drachenberg CB, Papadimitriou JC.Isolated visceral leishmaniasis presenting as an adrenal cystic mass. Archives of Pathology & Laboratory Medicine. 2000;**124**:1553–1556

[41] Teixeira Vde P, Hial V, Gomes RA, Castro EC, Reis M das G, Rodrigues ML, et al. Correlation between adrenal central vein parasitism and heart fibrosis in chronic chagasic myocarditis. The American Journal of Tropical Medicine and Hygiene. 1997;**56**:177–180

[42] Reincke M, Arlt W, Heppner C, Petzke F, Chrousos GP, Allolio B. Neuroendocrine dysfunction in african trypanosomiasis: The role of cytokinesa. Annals of the New York Academy of Sciences. 1998;**840**:809–821

[43] Pinto AY, Valente Vda C, Coura JR, Valente SA, Junqueira AC, Santos LC, et al. Clinical follow-up of responses to treatment with benznidazol in Amazon: A cohort study of acute chagas disease. PLoS One. 2013;**8**:e64450

[44] Mertens RB, Didier ES, Fishbein MC, Bertucci DC, Rogers LB, Orenstein JM. Encephalitozoon cuniculi microsporidiosis: Infection of the brain, heart, kidneys, trachea, adrenal glands, and urinary bladder in a patient with AIDS. Modern Pathology. 1997;**10**:68–77

[45] Mastorakos G, MAGIAKOU MA, Chrousos GP. Effects of the immune/inflammatory reaction on the hypothalamic-pituitary-adrenal axis. Annals of the New York Academy of Sciences. 1995;**771**:438–448

[46] Grulich AE, Li Y, McDonald AM, Correll PK, Law MG, Kaldor JM. Decreasing rates of Kaposi's sarcoma and non-Hodgkin's lymphoma in the era of potent combination anti-retroviral therapy. Aids. 2001;**15**:629–633

[47] Meher D, Duttab D, Giric R, Kard M. Adrenal leiomyoma mimicking adrenal malignancy: Diagnostic challenges and review of literature. Journal of Endocrinology and Metabolism. 2015;**5**:304–308

[48] Alteer M, Ascott-Evans BH, Conradie M. Leiomyoma: A rare cause of adrenal incidentaloma. JEMDSA. 2013;**18**:71–74

[49] Kumar S, Nanjappa B, Agrawal P, Pushkarna A. Large bilateral adrenal leiomyomas presenting as calcified adrenal masses: A rare case report. Korean Journal of Urology. 2014;**55**:363–366

[50] Dahan H, Bèges C, Weiss L, Abitbol M, Ledreff O, Teman G, et al. Leiomyoma of the adrenal gland in a patient with AIDS. Abdominal Imaging. 1994;**19**:259–261

[51] Radin DR, Kiyabu M. Multiple smooth-muscle tumours of the colon and adrenal gland in an adult with AIDS. American Journal of Roentgenology. 1992;**159**:545–546

[52] Lin J, Wasco MJ, Korobkin M, Doherty G, Giordano TJ. Leiomyoma of the adrenal gland presenting as a non-functioning adrenal incidentaloma: Case report and review of the literature. Endocrine Pathology. 2007;**18**:239–243

[53] Day DL, Sane S, Dehner LP. Inflammatory pseudotumor of the mesentery and small intestine. Pediatric Radiology. 1986;**16**:210–215. DOI: 10.1007/BF02456289

[54] Brunn H. Two interesting benign lung tumours of contradictory histopathology: Remarks on the necessity for maintaining the chest tumour registry. The Journal of Thoracic and Cardiovascular Surgery. 1939;**9**:119–131

[55] Umiker WO, Iverson L. Postinflammatory 'tumours' of the lung: report of four cases simulating xanthoma, fibroma, or plasma cell tumour. The Journal of Thoracic and Cardiovascular Surgery. 1954;**28**:55–63

[56] Sastre-Garau X, Couturier J, Derré J, Aurias A, Klijanienko J, Lagacé R. Inflammatory myofibroblastic tumour (inflammatory pseudotumour) of the breast. Clinicopathological and genetic analysis of a case with evidence for clonality. The Journal of Pathology. 2002;**196**(1):97–102. DOI: 10.1002/path.1004

[57] Pettinato G, Manivel JC, De Rosa N, Dehner LP. Inflammatory myofibroblastic tumor (plasma cell granuloma). Clinicopathologic study of 20 cases with immunohistochemical and ultrastructural observations. American Journal of Clinical Pathology. 1990;**94**(5):538–546

[58] Materne R, Van Beers BE, Gigot JF, et al. Inflammatory pseudotumor of the liver: MRI with mangafodipir trisodium. Journal of Computer Assisted Tomography. 1998;**22**:82–84

[59] Chawla A, Hameed Z, Mishra D, Monappa V. Adrenal inflammatory myofibroblastic tumour. BMJ Case Reports. 2013. DOI: 10.1136/bcr-2013-010122

[60] Tran-Dang M-A, Banga N, Khoo B, Bates AW. Inflammatory myofibroblastic tumour arising in the adrenal gland: A case report. Journal of Medical Case Reports. 2014;**8**:411. DOI: 10.1186/1752-1947-8-411

[61] Abehsera M, Vilgrain V, Belghiti J, Fléjou JF, Nahum H. Inflammatory pseudotumor of the liver: Radiologic—pathologic correlation. Journal of Computer Assisted Tomography. 1995;**19**:80–83

[62] Marino-Enriquez A, Wang WL, Roy A, Lopez-Terrada D, Lazar AJ, Fletcher CD, et al. Epithelioid inflammatory myofibroblastic sarcoma; an aggressive intra-abdominal variant of inflammatory myofibroblastic tumour with nuclear membrane or perinuclear ALK. The American Journal of Surgical Pathology. 2011;**35**:135–144. DOI: 10.1097/PAS.0b013e318200cfd5

[63] Attili SV, Chandra CR, Hemant DK, Bapsy PP, RamaRao C, Anupama G. Retroperitoneal inflammatory myofibroblastic tumor. World Journal of Surgical Oncology. 2005;**3**:66. DOI: 10.1186/1477-7819-3-66

[64] Coffin CM, Hornick JL, Fletcher CDM. Inflammatory myofibroblastic tumour; comparison of clinicopathologic, histologic, immunohistochemical features and ALK expression in atypical and aggressive cases. The American Journal of Surgical Pathology. 2007;**31**:509–520. DOI: 10.1097/01.pas.0000213393.57322.c7

[65] Stout AP. A tumor of the ulnar nerve. Proc NY Pathol Soc. 1918;**12**:2–12

[66] Hart MN, Earle KM. Primitive neuroectodermal tumors of the brain in children. Cancer. 1973;**32**:890–897

[67] Zhang Y, Li H. Primitive neuroectodermal tumors of adrenal gland. Japanese Journal of Clinical Oncology 2010;**40**:800–804

[68] Khong PL, Chan GC, Shek TW, Tam PK, Chan FL. Imaging of peripheral PNET: Common and uncommon locations. Clinical Radiology. 2002;**57**:272–277

[69] Rossi S, Orvieto E, Furlanetto A, Laurino L, Ninfo V, Dei Tos AP. Utility of the immunohistochemical detection of FLI-1 expression in round cell and vascular neoplasm using a monoclonal antibody. Modern Pathology. 2004;**17**:547–552

[70] Dutta D, Shivaprasad KS, Das RN, Ghosh S, Chowdhury S. Primitive neuroectodermal tumor of adrenal: Clinical presentation and outcomes. Journal of Cancer Research and Therapeutics. 2013;**9**:709–711. DOI: 10.4103/0973-1482.126459

[71] Fellinger EJ, Garin-Chesa P, Triche TJ, Huvos AG, Rettig WJ. Immunohistochemical analysis of Ewing's sarcoma cell surface antigen p30/32MIC2. American Journal of Pathology. 1991;**139**:317–325

[72] Weidner N, Tjoe J. Immunohistochemical profile of monoclonal antibody O13: antibody that recognizes glycoprotein p30/32MIC2 and is useful in diagnosing Ewing's sarcoma and peripheral neuroepithelioma. The American Journal of Surgical Pathology. 1994;**18**:486–494

[73] Komatsu S, Watanabe R, Naito M, Mizusawa T, Obara K, Nishiyama T, et al. Primitive neuroectodermal tumor of the adrenal gland. International Journal of Urology. 2006;**13**: 606–607

[74] Tsang YP, Lang BHH, Tam SC, Wong KP. Primitive neuroectodermal adrenal gland tumour. Hong Kong Medical Journal. 2014;**20**:444–446

[75] Phukan C, Nirmal TJ, Kumar RM, Kekre NS. Peripheral primitive neuroectodermal tumor of the adrenal gland: A rare entity. Indian Journal of Urology : IJU : Journal of the Urological Society of India. 2013;**29**:357–359. DOI: 10.4103/0970-1591.120128

[76] Wong DD, Spagnolo DV, Bisceglia M, Havlat M, McCallum D, Platten MA. Oncocytic adrenocortical neoplasms—A clinicopathologic study of 13 new cases emphasizing the importance of their recognition. Human Pathology. 2011;**42**:489–499. DOI: 10.1016/j.humpath.2010.08.010

[77] Sharma N, Dogra PN, Mathur S. Functional adrenal oncocytoma: A rare neoplasm. Indian Journal of Pathology and Microbiology. 2008;**51**:531–533

[78] Alexander A, Paulose KP. Oncocytic variant of adrenal carcinoma presenting as Cushing's syndrome. The Journal of the Association of Physicians of India. 1998;**46**:235–237

[79] Mearini L, Sordo RD, Costantini E, Nunzi E, Porena M. Adrenal oncocytic neoplasm: A systematic review. Urologia Internationalis. 2013;**91**:125–133. DOI: 10.1159/000345141

[80] Bisceglia M, Ludovico O, Mattia AD, Ben-Dor D, Sandbank J, Pasquinelli G, et al. Adrenocortical oncocytic tumors: Report of 10 cases and review of the literature. International Journal of Surgical Pathology. 2004;**12**:231–243

[81] Shah VN, Premkumar A, Walia R, Kumar S, Nahar U, Bhansali A. Large but benign adrenal mass: Adrenal oncocytoma. Indian Journal of Endocrinology and Metabolism. 2012;**16**:469–471. DOI: 10.4103/2230-8210.95717

[82] Schittenhelm J, Ebner FH, Harter P, Bornemann A. Symptomatic intraspinal oncocytic adrenocortical adenoma. Endocrine Pathology. 2009;**20**:73–77. DOI: 10.1007/s12022-008-9051-1

[83] Ciancio G, Vaidya A, Shirodkar S, Manoharan M, Hakky T, Soloway M. En bloc mobilization of the pancreas and spleen to facilitate resection of large tumors, primarily renal and adrenal, in the left upper quadrant of the abdomen: Techniques derived from multivisceral transplantation. European Urology. 2009;**55**:1106–1111. DOI: 10.1016/j.eururo.2008.12.038

[84] Kumar S, Jayant K, Prasad S, Agrawal S, Parmar KM, Roat R, et al. Rare adrenal gland emergencies: A case series of giant myelolipoma presenting with massive hemorrhage and abscess. Nephro-Urology Monthly. Jan 2015;**7**(1):e22671

[85] Kenney PJ, Wagner BJ, Rao P, Heffess CS. Myelolipoma: CT and pathologic features. Radiology. 1998;**208**:87–95. DOI: 10.1148/radiology.208.1.9646797

[86] Lee JK. Computed Body Tomography with MRI Correlation. Lippincott Williams & Wilkins; 2006 ISBN: 0781745268

[87] Gamss C, Chia F, Chernyak V, Rozenblit A. Giant hemorrhagic myelolipoma in a patient with sickle cell disease. Emergency Radiology. 2009;**16**:319–322. DOI: 10.1007/s10140-008-0740-3

[88] Kamani F, Mohammadi SS, Hessami R, Rezvani N, Peirovi H, Tavassoli S. Giant adrenal myelolipoma associated with beta-thalassemia: A case report. International Journal of Endocrinology and Metabolism. 2009;**7**:259–262

[89] Civrilli K, Damry N, Steppe R, Efira A, Mathieu J. Bilateral adrenal myelolipomas. JBR-BTR. 2008;**91**:90–91

[90] Bishop E, Eble JN, Cheng L, Wang M, Chase DR, Orazi A, O'Malley DP. Adrenal myelolipomas show nonrandom X-chromosome inactivation in hematopoietic elements and fat: Support for a clonal origin of myelolipomas. The American Journal of Surgical Pathology. 2006;**30**:838–843

[91] Chang KC, Chen PI, Huang ZH, Lin YM, Kuo PL. Adrenal myelolipoma with translocation (3;21)(q25; p11). Cancer Genetics and Cytogenetics. 2002;**134**:77–80

[92] Han M, Burnett AL, Fishman EK, et al. The natural history and treatment of adrenal myelolipoma. Journal of Urology. 1997;**157**:1213–1216

[93] Meyer A, Behrend M. Presentation and therapy of myelolipoma. International Journal of Urology. 2005;**12**:239–243. DOI: 10.1111/j.1442-2042.2005.01034.x

[94] Russell C, Goodacre BW, vanSonnenberg E, Orihuela E. Spontaneous rupture of adrenal myelolipoma: Spiral CT appearance. Abdominal Imaging. 2000;**25**:431–434

[95] Behrend M, Kaaden S, von Wasielewski R, Frericks B. Benign retroperitoneal schwannoma mimicking an adrenal mass. Surgical Laparoscopy Endoscopy & Percutaneous Techniques. 2003;**13**:133–138

[96] Korets R, Berkenblit R, Ghavamian R. Incidentally Discovered Adrenal Schwannoma. JSLS. 2007;**11**:113–115

[97] Adas M, Ozulker F, Adas G, Koc B, Ozulker T, Sahin IM. A rare adrenal incidentaloma: Adrenal schwannoma. Case Reports in Gastroenterology. 2013;**7**:420–427

[98] Lau SK, Spagnolo DV, Weiss LM. Schwannoma of the adrenal gland: Report of two cases. The American Journal of Surgical Pathology. 2006;**30**:630–634

[99] Târcoveanu E, Dimofte G, Bradea C, Moldovanu R, Vasilescu A, Anton R, Ferariu D. Adrenal schwannoma. JSLS. 2009;**13**:116–119

[100] Onoda N, Ishikawa T, Toyokawa T, Takashima T, Wakasa K, Hirakawa K. Adrenal schwannoma treated with laparoscopic surgery. JSLS. 2008;**12**:420–425

[101] Tenenbaum F, Groussin L, Foehrenbach H, Tissier F, Gouya H, Bertherat J, Dousset B, Legmann P, Richard B, Bertagna X. 18F–fluorodeoxyglucose positron emission tomography as a diagnostic tool for malignancy of adrenocortical tumours? Preliminary results in 13 consecutive patients. European Journal of Endocrinology. 2004;**150**:789–792

[102] Fine SW, McClain SA, Li M. Immunohistochemical staining for calretinin is useful for differentiating schwannomas from neurofibromas. American Journal of Clinical Pathology. 2004;**122**:552–559

[103] Nishio A, Adachi W, Igarashi J, Koide N, Kajikawa S, Amano J. Laparoscopic resection of a retroperitoneal schwannoma. Surgical Laparoscopy Endoscopy & Percutaneous Techniques. 1999;**9**:306–309

[104] Enzinger F, Weiss S. Primitive neuroectodermal tumors and related lesions. Soft Tissue Tumors. St. Louis: Mosby; 1995. pp. 929–964

[105] Radin R, David CL, Goldfarb H, Francis IR. Adrenal and extra-adrenal retroperitoneal ganglioneuroma: imaging findings in 13 adults. Radiology. 1997;**202**:703–707

[106] Majbar AM, Elmouhadi S, Elaloui M, Raiss M, Sabbah F, Hrora A, et al. Imaging features of adrenal ganglioneuroma: A case report. BMC Research Notes. 2014;**7**:791

[107] Kumar S, Singh S, Chandna A. Organ Preservation in a Case of Retroperitoneal Ganglioneuroma. Case Reports in Surgery. Accepted 17 August 2016. Ahead of print. http://www.hindawi.com/journals/cris/aip/6597374/

[108] Jain D, Chopra P, Sharma A. Adrenal lipoma with hemorrhage. Urology Journal. 2012;**9**:721–724

[109] Lam KY, Lo CY. Adrenal lipomatous tumours: A 30 year clinicopathological experience at a single institution. Journal of Clinical Pathology. 2001;**54**:707–712

[110] Milathianakis KN, Farfarelos CD, Mpogdanos IM, Karamanolakis DK. Giant lipoma of the adrenal gland. Journal of Urology. 2002;**167**:1777

[111] Singaporewalla RM, Thamboo TP, Rau A, Cheah WK, Mukherjee JJ. Acute abdominal pain secondary to retrop- eritoneal bleeding from a giant adrenal lipoma with review of literature. Asian Journal of Surgery. 2009;**32**:172–176

[112] Shumaker N, Rochman C, Legallo R, Northup C, Hanks J. Incidentally identified adrenal lipoma: Case report and review of related literature. Endocrine Practice. 2008;**14**:209–212

[113] Lam KY, Chan AC, Ng IO. Giant adrenal lipoma: A report of two cases and review of literature. Scandinavian Journal of Urology. 1997;**31**:89–90

[114] Grumbach MM, Biller BM, Braunstein GD, Campbell KK, Carney JA, Godley PA, et al. Management of the clinically inapparent adrenal mass ("incidentaloma"). Annals of Internal Medicine. 2003;**138**:424–429

[115] Andreoni C, Krebs RK, Bruna PC, Goldman SM, Kater CE, Alves MT, et al. Cystic phaeochromocytoma is a distinctive subgroup with special clinical, imaging and histological features that might mislead the diagnosis. BJU International. 2008;**101**:345–350

[116] Erem C, Kocak M, OnderErsoz H, Ersoz S, Yucel Y. Epinephrine-secreting cystic pheochromocytoma presenting with an incidental adrenal mass: A case report and a review of the literature. Endocrine. 2005;**28**:225–230

[117] Takarabea D, Takahashib Y, Tsujimotoa T, Notoa H, Kishimotoa M, Minowadad S, et al. Cystic pheochromocytoma discovered as an adrenal incidentaloma. Journal of Medical Cases. 2013;**11**:753–757

[118] Wang H, Sun B, Xu Z, Lei W, Wang X. Undiagnosed giant cystic pheochromocytoma: A case report. Oncology Letters. 2015;**10**:1444–1446. http://dx.doi.org/10.3892/ol.2015.3484

[119] Rogers CG, Pinto PA, Weir EG. Extraosseous (Extramedullary) Plasmacytoma of the adrenal gland. Archives of Pathology & Laboratory Medicine. 2004;**128**:e86-e88

[120] Soutar R, Lucraft H, Jackson G, Reece A, Bird J, Low E, et al. Guidelines on the diagnosis and management of solitary plasmacytoma of bone and solitary extramedullary plasmacytoma. Clinical Oncology. 2004;**16**:405–413

[121] Cao D, Li L, Liu L, Xiao W, He X, Tang Z, et al. Solitary extramedullary plasmacytoma of the adrenal gland: A rare case report with review of the literature. International Journal of Clinical and Experimental Pathology. 2014;**7**:9072–9075

[122] Pasch W, Zhao XH, Pezk SA. Solitary plasmacytoma of the bone involving young individuals, is there a role for preceding trauma?. International Journal of Clinical and Experimental Pathology. 2012;**5**:463–467

[123] Bhattacharya AK, Han K, Baredes S. Extramedullary plasmacytoma of the head and neck associated with the human immunodeficiency virus. Ear, Nose & Throat Journal. 1998;**77**:61–62

[124] Fujikata S, Tanji N, Aoki K, Ohoka H, Hojo N, Yokoyama M. Extramedullary plasmacytoma arising from an adrenal gland. Urology. 2002;**60**:514v-514. viii

[125] Ahmed M, Al-Ghamdi A, Al-Omari M, Aljurf M, Al-Kadhi Y. Autologous bone marrow transplanation for extramedullary plasmacytoma presenting as adrenal incidentaloma. Annals of Saudi Medicine. 2009;**29**:219–222. DOI: 10.4103/0256-4947.51785

[126] Khurana A, Kaur P, Chauhan AK, Kataria SP, Bansal N. Primary non Hodgkin's lymphoma of left adrenal gland—A rare presentation. Journal of Clinical and Diagnostic Research. 2015;**9**:XD01-XD03. DOI: 10.7860/JCDR/2015/8079.5745

[127] Freeman C, Berg JW, Culter SJ. Occurrence and prognosis of extranodal lymphomas. Cancer. 1972;**29**:252–260

[128] Sachico IW, Tohru A, Nayoyoshi M. Bilateral adrenal lymphoma with hypercalcemia: An autopsy case report with a review of the literature. Journal of Clinical and Experimental Hematopathology. 2003;**51**:101–109

[129] Simpson WG, Babbar P, Payne LF. Bilateral primary adrenal non-Hodgkin's lymphoma without adrenal insufficiency. Urology Annals. 2015;**7**:259–261. DOI: 10.4103/0974-7796.152942

[130] Cavanna L, Civardi G, Vallisa D, Bertè R. Primary adrenal non-Hodgkin's lymphoma associated with autoimmune hemolytic anemia: A case diagnosed by ultrasound-guided fine needle biopsy. Annali italiani di medicina interna. 1999;**14**(4):298–301

[131] Edwards JP, Stuart HC, Urbanski SJ, Pasieka JL. A rare cavernous hemangioma of the adrenal gland. International Journal of Surgery Case Reports. 2014;**5**:52–55. DOI: 10.1016/j.ijscr.2013.11.003

[132] Abou El-Ghar M, Refaie H, El-Hefnawy A, El-Diasty T. Adrenal hemangioma: Findings at multidetector CT with short review of the literature. Case Reports in Radiology. 2011;**2011**:601803

[133] Forbes TL. Retroperitoneal hemorrhage secondary to a ruptured cavernous hemangioma. Canadian Journal of Surgery. 2005;**48**:78–79

[134] Auh YH, Anand J, Zirinsky K, Kazam E. Adrenal hemangioma: A case report. Journal of Computer Assisted Tomography. 1986;**10**:57–59

[135] Boraschi P, Campatelli A, Di Vito A, Perri G. Hemorrhage in cavernous hemangioma of the adrenal gland: US, CT and MRI appearances with pathologic correlation. European Journal of Radiology. 1995;**21**:41–43

[136] Yamada T, Ishibashi T, Saito H, Majima K, Tsuda M, Takahashi S, et al. Two cases of adrenal hemangioma: CT and MRI findings with pathological correlations. Radiation Medicine. 2002;**20**:51–56

[137] Deckers F, De Schepper A, Shamsi K, Hauben E, Van March E. Cavernous hemangioma of the adrenal gland: CT appearance. Journal of Computer Assisted Tomography. 1993;**17**:506–507

[138] Kumar S, Mandal AK, Acharya N, Thingnam SK, Bhalla V, Singh SK. Superior mesenteric artery injury during en bloc excision of a massive left adrenal Tumor. Urologia Internationalis 2007;**78**:182–184. DOI: 10.1159/000098081

Chapter 3

Pheochromocytomas and Paragangliomas: A Focus on Genetics

Diana Loreta Păun and Alexandra Mirică

Additional information is available at the end of the chapter

http://dx.doi.org/10.5772/67374

Abstract

Pheochromocytomas and paragangliomas are rare tumors, characterized by catecholamine synthesis, release, and metabolism, with the same embryological origin. Pheochromocytomas develop from chromaffin cells of the adrenal medulla, whereas paragangliomas arise extra-adrenal from sympathetic and parasympathetic nervous chains. During the past 10 years, there have been significant advances in the understanding of these tumors as it is now known that 30–40% of pheochromocytomas and paragangliomas have an underlying genetic cause. Pheochromocytomas and paragangliomas have classically been associated with three syndromes: von Hippel-Lindau (VHL), multiple endocrine neoplasia type 2 (MEN 2), and neurofibromatosis type 1 (NF1). To date, more than 21 gene mutations have been identified that are involved in the development of these tumors. Identification of such gene mutations associated with pheochromocytomas and paragangliomas will ensure early diagnosis, prompt treatment, and better prognosis for patient and family members. The recent developments in molecular pathogenesis of pheochromocytomas and paragangliomas will provide future treatment options toward personalized therapy for patients. This chapter summarizes the most important aspects of genetics and clinical characteristics, together with a focus on the new susceptibility genes.

Keywords: genetics, pheochromocytomas, paragangliomas, susceptibility genes

1. Introduction

The tumor classification system by the World Health Organization (WHO) in 2004 defines pheochromocytomas as catecholamine-secreting tumors originating from chromaffin cells found in the medulla of adrenal glands, and paragangliomas as extra-adrenal tumors developing from ganglia along the sympathetic and parasympathetic autonomic nervous chains [1]. Head and neck paragangliomas (formerly, called glomus tumors) are derived from parasympathetic paraganglia, arising in the vagal and carotid bodies, jugulotympanic region (middle ear), orbit, or nasal cavity. They are nonchromaffin tumors (negative staining to chromium salts) and usually nonfunctional with the exception of a minority of these tumors (20–30%) that produce mostly methoxytyramine [2, 3]. Head and neck paragangliomas demonstrate usually a slow growth rate benign in nature with symptoms dependent on their location. As a result, they can cause clinical signs of compression and infiltration of adjacent neurovascular structures, such as cranial nerve palsy, hearing loss, and tinnitus [4].

Sympathetic paragangliomas are found in the mediastinum (from the thoracic sympathetic nervous chain), pre- and paravertebral autonomic nervous chains and para-aortic sympathetic chains of the thorax, abdomen, and pelvis, including the organ of Zuckerkandl. These tumors often secrete catecholamines, especially norepinephrine, and are chromaffin-positive tumors. Due to their catecholamine secretory profile, pheochromocytomas and sympathetic paragangliomas can share the same clinical symptoms with the "the classic triad" of palpitations, diaphoresis, and headache. Clinical signs can appear suddenly or be precipitated by physical activity, drugs (e.g. metoclopramide and glucocorticoids), foods containing tyramine, diagnostic procedures, or micturition [5].

Pheochromocytomas and paragangliomas affect about 1 in 2500–6500 persons, but this incidence may be more significant because of this disease diagnosis made after the person's death [6]. Pheochromocytomas are found in approximately 4–5% of adrenal incidentalomas, and together with sympathetic paragangliomas, can be a secondary cause of hypertension in about 0.2–0.4% of the cases [7]. Paragangliomas can appear in all ages, but their highest incidence is between 40 and 50 years with no sex differences.

Although mostly benign, 10–15% of such tumors are malignant, consisting of metastatic spread of chromaffin cells especially in the liver, lungs, bone, and lymph nodes [8]. Despite much investigation, no definite biochemical, genetic, or histological markers to determine the malignant character of these particular neuroendocrine tumors has been identified. In this regard, the Pheochromocytoma of the Adrenal Gland Scaled Score (PASS) was created to predict the malignant character of pheochromocytomas with a PASS score of <4 suggesting benignity, whereas a PASS score >4 indicating a potentially malignant tumor [9]. Nevertheless, a large retrospective study indicated no correlation of predictive risk and PASS score for malignancy [10]. Moreover, Ki-67 index of proliferation used commonly as a marker of malignancy in other tumors demonstrated no utility for distinguishing between benign or malignant pheochromocytomas and paragangliomas [11]. In addition, studies have revealed certain factors that predict malignancy for pheochromocytomas and paragangliomas: the extra-adrenal tumors in the mediastinum or the organ of Zuckerkandl, tumor size >5 cm, increased expression of angiogenesis-related genes by immunohistochemistry, increased plasmatic levels of 3-methoxytyramine or chromogranin A, younger age at diagnosis, and identification of a SDHB mutation [12–15]. This chapter summarizes recent data regarding pheochromocytomas and paragangliomas with a focus on genetics. Furthermore, a genetic testing algorithm is proposed for the clinical management of such patients with these tumors.

2. Genetics of pheochromocytomas and paragangliomas

Before 2000, pheochromocytomas and paragangliomas were thought to follow the 10% rule: 10% familial, 10% bilateral, 10% extra-adrenal, 10% malignant, 10% children, 10% not hypertensive, and 10% calcified. It was previously believed that familial pheochromocytomas and paragangliomas were caused by three gene mutations that determined three distinct clinical syndromes: multiple endocrine neoplasia type 2 (MEN2) syndrome involving RET proto-oncogene mutations, neurofibromatosis type I caused by NF1 gene mutations and von Hippel-Lindau disease produced by VHL gene mutations. Recent studies, however, reveal that 30–40% from pheochromocytomas and paragangliomas have an underlying genetic pathogenesis, and some sporadic tumors are caused by somatic mutations in 10–24% of the cases [16, 17].

Currently, more than 21 genes (RET, NF1, VHL, SDHA, SDHB, SDHC, SDHD, SDHAF2, MAX, TMEM127, HIF2A, KIF1Bβ, H-RAS, K-RAS, PHD2/EGLN1, IDH, ATRX, MDH2, PHD1, FH, and BAP1) are known to cause hereditary pheochromocytomas and paragangliomas. By the main signaling pathways, these genes have been grouped into two clusters:

1. Cluster 1, a pseudohypoxic group, referring to mutations in VHL, HIF2A, SDHx, EGLN1/PHD2, IDH, MDH2, and FH genes
2. Cluster 2, a kinase receptor-signaling group of genes, involving mutations in NF1, RET, MAX, TMEM127, and KIF1B genes.

Recent studies have demonstrated that the two clusters are connected by particular signaling pathways, all leading to tumorigenesis of pheochromocytomas and paragangliomas [18]. This elevated percentage of tumors with molecular pathogenesis indicates genetic testing as a mandatory step in the clinical management of patients with pheochromocytomas and paragangliomas.

2.1. Syndromic tumors

2.1.1. RET proto-oncogene

The REarranged during Transfection (RET) proto-oncogene is located on chromosome 10, and its translated protein is a transmembrane receptor from the tyrosine kinase family that controls cellular growth, differentiation, and apoptosis. Germline mutation of RET activates this RET receptor with "gain of function." This activation consequently leads to cell proliferation, causing an autosomal-dominant syndrome called multiple endocrine neoplasia type 2 (MEN2). This syndrome is classified into two subcategories: MEN2A and MEN2B. MEN2A syndrome is further divided in four types: classical MEN2A, MEN2A associated with cutaneous lichen amyloidosis, MEN2A associated with Hirschprung's disease, and familial medullary thyroid cancer (FMTC).

The classical form of MEN2A syndrome is most frequent, occurring in approximately 90% of cases. It is characterized by medullary thyroid carcinoma (MTC) in 95% of cases, pheochromocytoma in 50% of cases and hyperparathyroidism in 15–30% of cases. FMTC is represented by this thyroid cancer as the only clinical feature [5]. MEN2B syndrome is composed of MTC in all the cases, and pheochromocytoma in half of patients together with intestinal ganglioneuromas, multiple mucosal neuromas, and marfanoid habitus.

The MEN2 subcategories are linked with the RET gene defects. Most mutations of the RET gene in MEN2A and FMTC patients involve codons: 609, 611, 618, 620 (exon 10) or 630, and 634 (exon 11). The mutation at codon 634, consisting in a majority of cases in the substitution of the amino acid cysteine to arginine, is the most frequent genetic defect in patients with MEN2A syndrome who have a high risk of pheochromocytoma. Regarding MEN2B, the majority of cases are determined by the codon 918 mutation (exon 16), leading to the substitution of methionine to threonine. Additionally, rare mutations in codon exon 14 and 15 have been associated with this type of MEN2 [19].

Pheochromocytomas associated with MEN2A and MEN2B syndromes are frequently benign and bilateral in a majority of cases at a young age diagnosed between 30 and 40 years. The malignancy rate is less than 1–5%. The secretory profile is characterized by hypersecretion of epinephrine, caused by the overexpression of phenylethanolamine-N-methyltransferase [16].

2.1.2. Neurofibromatosis type 1 tumor suppressor gene

Neurofibromatosis type 1 (NF1) syndrome, also called von Recklinghausen's disease, is an autosomal dominant condition caused by mutations of the large neurofibromatosis type 1 tumor suppressor gene (NF1). This gene is located on chromosome 17q11.2 and encodes for the protein neurofibromin, which enters nervous cells (e.g., neurons, Schwann cells, and oligodendrocytes), leukocytes, keratinocytes, and adrenal medulla [5].

NF1 gene defects can cause the inhibition of RAS signaling cascade, acceleration of phosphoinositide 3-kinase (PI3K), mitogen-activated protein kinase (MAPK), and mammalian target of rapamycin (mTOR) pathways. As a result, NF1 defects play a role in the alteration of cell growth, differentiation, migration, and apoptosis. Nevertheless, more than a half of NF1 patients present *de novo* defects of the NF1 gene. Diagnosis of NF1 is based on clinical criteria (at least two): six or more café- au- lait spots, two or more iris hamartomas (Lisch nodules), two or more cutaneous neurofibromas, optic-nerve glioma, freckling in the axilla, neck, or inguinal, pseudoarthrosis or dysplasia of the sphenoid bone, and a first-degree family member with a diagnosis of NF1.

Patients with NF1 also have an increased risk for brainstem gliomas, astrocytomas, gastrointestinal stromal tumors, rhabdomyosarcomas, chronic myeloid leukemias, and pheochromocytomas. The incidence of pheochromocytomas in NF1 patients is approximately 0.1–5.7%, typically by 42 years of age. Cases of sympathetic paragangliomas are very rarely reported. Most pheochromocytomas are unilateral, benign, and have an epinephrine secretory profile. The rate of malignancy for pheochromocytomas in NF1 patients is approximately 12%, a little higher than in MEN2, and VHL patients [20, 21].

2.1.3. Von Hippel-Lindau disease tumor suppressor gene

Von Hippel-Lindau (VHL) tumor suppressor gene is located on the short arm of chromosome 3, and this gene encodes for VHL protein that controls the actions of hypoxia-inducible factor alpha (HIFα). Germline mutations of this tumor suppressor gene cause VHL disease, an autosomal dominant disorder that comprises a large variety of tumors: retinal angiomas, cerebellar and spinal hemangioblastomas, clear cell renal carcinoma, neuroendocrine tumors of the pancreas, epididymal cystadenomas, cysts of the broad ligament, endolymphatic sac tumors, pheochromocytomas, and paragangliomas. Depending on the presence of pheochromocytomas and paragangliomas, VHL disease is divided into type 1 and type 2. Type 1 VHL disease is the most common form, characterized by the absence of pheochromocytomas and paragangliomas. Conversely, type 2 VHL disease is distinguished by the development of pheochromocytomas and paragangliomas. Type 2 VHL disease is further classified into three subcategories: 2A without clear renal cell carcinoma, 2B with clear renal cell carcinoma, and 2C with only pheochromocytomas and paragangliomas [16].

VHL gene mutations are variable, and >500 germline transformations have been described (i.e., insertions, deletions, missense, nonsense, and splice site mutations) with a rate of occurrence of *de novo* mutations of up to 20%. In type 1 VHL disease, the most frequently encountered are deletions and nonsense mutations, whereas in type 2 VHL diseases, the most common are missense mutations. It is important to note that missense mutations in codon 167 increase patient's risk to develop pheochromocytomas.

Sympathetic head and neck paragangliomas cases are rarely reported. Pheochromocytomas develop in 10–20% of VHL patients, more than a half of them being bilateral, with a young age of onset around 30 years. Pheochromocytomas and paragangliomas within this disorder secrete mainly norepinephrine due to the absence of the phenylethanolamine N-methyltransferase. Furthermore, malignant pheochromocytomas have been reported in few cases, lower than 5% of VHL patients [22].

2.1.4. Genes encoding succinate dehydrogenase mitochondrial complex

Gene mutations encoding for the succinate dehydrogenase (SDH) complex (SDHA, SDHB, SDHC, SDHD, and the cofactor SDHAF2) lead to clinical manifestations of the familial paraganglioma (PGL) syndromes (PGL1, PGL2, PGL3, and PGL4). The SDH complex plays a role in the Krebs cycle and electron transport chain, and its genetic defects effect the increase of succinate and reactive oxygen species and stabilization of hypoxia-inducible factor 1 (HIF-1). Mutations of the SDH complex resemble VHL disease where the hypoxia signaling pathways are activated [23].

2.1.4.1. PGL 1 syndrome

Paraganglioma 1 (PGL1) syndrome is an autosomal-dominant condition, with maternal imprinting, caused by SDHD gene defects. This particular gene is localized on the long arm of chromosome 11. The clinical characteristics of this syndrome are multifocal nonsecretory parasympathetic head and neck paragangliomas and, less commonly, sympathetic thoracic or abdominal paragangliomas. Furthermore, pheochromocytomas have rarely been described. Tumor malignant transformation for SDHD mutation carriers is <5% [24].

2.1.4.2. PGL 2 syndrome

Familial paraganglioma 2 (PGL2) syndrome is a rare autosomal-dominant transmitted condition, with maternal imprinting, caused by genetic defects in SDHAF2/SDH5 gene that is localized on the long arm of chromosome 11. The gene product is succinate dehydrogenase assembly factor 2 (SDHAF2), which ensures the flavination of SDHA subunit. Studies have reported that mutations carriers have exclusively multifocal head and neck paragangliomas with an early onset from 30 to 40 years [25].

2.1.4.3. PGL 3 syndrome

Familial paraganglioma 3 (PGL3) syndrome, also with an autosomal dominant mode of transmission, is caused by SDHC gene mutations that are localized on the long arm of chromosome 1. This disorder is characterized by the presence of benign parasympathetic head and neck in paragangliomas up to 4% of patients. However, few cases of pheochromocytomas and sympathetic paragangliomas have been described. The biochemical phenotype is frequently associated with noradrenergic or dopaminergic secretion, but they can also be nonsecreting tumors. The malignancy rate of these tumors is very low [26].

2.1.4.4. PGL 4 syndrome

The most frequently encountered modification, germline mutations of the SDHB gene found in locus 1 p36.13 cause familial paraganglioma 4 (PGL4) syndrome. The clinical manifestations of this disorder consist in thoracic, abdominal, and pelvic catecholamine-secreting paragangliomas, parasympathetic head and neck paragangliomas. Tumors associated with

SDHB gene mutations are frequently multiple, large, presenting a noradrenergic or dopaminergic secretory profile. Diagnosis is usually made at a young age (approximately 30 years), and they are linked to a high risk of developing metastases (ranging from 30 to 72% of cases). As a result, all patients with malignant pheochromocytomas and paragangliomas should undergo genetic screening, searching initially for SDHB gene modifications. Patients with PGL4 syndrome present a high risk for developing clear cell renal carcinoma, neuroblastoma, papillary thyroid carcinoma, breast neoplasms and gastrointestinal stromal tumors (GIST) [18, 21, 23, 27, 28].

SDHA gene mutations localized on the short arm of chromosome 5 which were initially found only in homozygous carriers, were linked to the rare juvenile encephalopathy recognized also as Leigh syndrome. Additionally, paragangliomas were described in the heterozygous carriers of the SDHA gene mutations, having a malignancy rate of 0–14%. [29]. Germline mutations of the SDHB, SDHC, and SDHD genes were also identified in the Carney-Stratakis dyad that consists of gastrointestinal stromal tumors (GIST) and paragangliomas, and the Carney triad, composed of paragangliomas, GIST, and pulmonary chondromas. The secretory profile of SDHx-related paragangliomas is characterized by an overproduction of norepinephrine together with dopamine, dopamine hypersecretion (or its metabolite 3-methoxytyramine) only, or a silent biochemical phenotype [5, 23, 30].

2.2. Nonsyndromic tumors

2.2.1. Other susceptibility genes

2.2.1.1. TMEM127 gene

The TMEM127 gene is localized on the long arm of chromosome 2, which encodes for transmembrane protein 127. Expression of this gene is associated with endosomes, lysosomes, and Golgi complex, acting as a negative factor of mTOR kinase pathways that modulates cell growth and apoptosis. Mutations of this gene induce the development of pheochromocytoma (unilateral or bilateral), abdominal and head and neck paragangliomas with adrenergic or noradrenergic biochemical phenotypes. Further studies report a 2% prevalence of TMEM127 germline mutations in patients with pheochromocytomas and paragangliomas at a mean age of 43 years. Risk for malignant transformation is approximately 1%. Other tumors such as breast and papillary thyroid carcinoma have been described in patients carrying this gene mutation [5, 18, 31, 32].

2.2.1.2. MAX gene

The MYC-associated factor X (MAX) gene localized on the short arm of chromosome 14 encodes for MAX protein, and its main role is in the modulation of cell growth and apoptosis as a component of the MYC-MAX-MXD1 complex. MAX gene germline defects have been described in patients with pheochromocytomas and paragangliomas. The tumors are frequently bilateral with a mean age of onset at 32 years. They also present with an increased malignant potential (25% of patients). Additionally, mutations of MAX gene have a paternal mode of transmission with maternal imprinting. They lead to the development of tumors with a norepinephrine secretory profile [5, 18, 33].

2.2.1.3. HIF2A gene

Hypoxia-inducible factor 2-alpha (HIF2A) gene mutations found in the locus 2p21 have recently been correlated with the development of pheochromocytomas and paragangliomas. HIF2A gene mutations determine a decreased rate of HIF2α protein degradation. They lead to an enhanced action of vascular endothelial growth factor A (VEGF-A) and erythropoietin that regulate cell proliferation, angiogenesis, and erythropoiesis. Somatic HIF2A gene mutations have been described in patients who presented with multiple pheochromocytomas and paragangliomas with a noradrenergic secretory profile, polycythemia, and somatostatinomas, which comprise the clinical features of the recently described Pacak-Zhuang syndrome. Of note, all patients with this syndrome were women, but further studies are required in order to establish the genetic basis [18, 34].

2.2.1.4. EGLN1/PHD2 gene

The egg-laying-defective nine 1 gene (EGLN1) also named prolyl hydroxylase domain 2 (PHD2) gene is located on chromosome 1q42.1, and encodes for the EGLN1/PHD2 protein that hydroxylates HIFα protein. Germline mutations of EGLN1/PHD2 gene have been associated with the development of multiple sympathetic abdominal paragangliomas and erythrocytosis [18, 35].

2.2.1.5. KIF1Bβ gene

The kinesin family 1Bβ gene (KIF1Bβ) is located on chromosome 1p36.22 and its product plays an important role in regulating cell apoptosis. Very rare cases of patients with germline KIF1B gene mutations have been reported to have unilateral or bilateral pheochromocytomas, neuroblastoma, ganglioneuroma, medulloblastoma, leiomyosarcoma, and lung adenocarcinoma [5, 18, 36].

2.2.1.6. IDH gene

The isocitrate dehydrogenase (IDH) gene is located on chromosome 2q33.3, and its mutations are frequently associated with glioblastoma multiforme. Studies conducted on patients with pheochromocytomas and paragangliomas indicate only one somatic mutation of the IDH gene associated in the development of carotid paragangliomas [18, 37].

2.2.1.7. FH gene

The fumarate hydratase (FH) gene is found on chromosome 1q43 and its germline mutation has been reported in one patient with a pheochromocytoma and noradrenergic secretory profile.

http://dx.doi.org/10.5772/67374

Furthermore, FH gene mutations have also been reported in patients with clear cell renal carcinoma and leiomyomatosis [11, 18, 38].

2.2.1.8. BAP1 gene

Germline mutations of BRCA-1 associated protein-1 (BAP1) gene located on chromosome 3p21.1 have been reported in a limited number of patients with paragangliomas. Moreover, BAP1 mutations were identified in some patients with meningioma, melanoma, and mesothelioma, but correlations with familial paragangliomas require further studies [18, 39].

2.2.1.9. HRAS and KRAS genes

The RAS genes (Harvey rat sarcoma—H-RAS virus gene located on chromosome 11p15, and Kirsten rat sarcoma virus gene—K RAS found on chromosome 12p12.1) are the most common oncogenes associated with malignancies. H-RAS and K-RAS gene mutations cause the constitutive activation of the GTPase domain of RAS, inducing cell growth through activated RAS-ERK (extracellular signal-regulated kinase) pathway. Somatic mutations in H-RAS and K-RAS have been described in limited cases of pheochromocytomas and paragangliomas with adrenergic or noradrenergic biochemical phenotype. Recently, one study regarding pheochromocytomas and paragangliomas stated that 6.9% of patients had somatic H-RAS mutations [40, 41].

2.2.2. Miscellaneous

One family with a germline mutation of Malate Dehydrogenase type 2 (MDH2) gene with multiple metastatic paragangliomas producing norepinephrine has been described [41, 42]. Furthermore, somatic mutations of Alpha Thalassemia/Mental Retardation Syndrome X-Linked (**ATRX)** gene have been described in aggressive cases of pheochromocytomas and paragangliomas. This gene, localized on the X chromosome, plays an important role in telomere function [41, 43]. Moreover, a novel germline mutation involving prolyl hydroxylase domain 1 (**PHD1)** also known as egg-laying-defective nine 2 gene (EGLN2) mutation was reported in one case of pheochromocytoma/paraganglioma, and polycythemia [41, 44].

Recent studies have also stated that the following genes play roles in the development of pheochromocytomas and paragangliomas: glial cell-derived neurotrophic factor (**GDNF**) localized on 5p13.2, guanine nucleotide binding protein (g protein) alpha stimulating (**GNAS**) found on 20q13.32, cyclin-dependent kinase inhibitor 2a (**CDKN2A**) localized on 9p21.3, breast cancers **BRCA 1 and 2** found on 17q21.31 and 13q13.1, respectively, lysine methyltransferase 2d (**KMT2D**) found on 12q13.12, and **tumor protein p53** localized on 17p13.1 [18, 46–48, 50].

All genes currently known to be involved in the pathogenesis of pheochromocytomas and paragangliomas, specifying the chromosomal location of the gene, hormonal secretory profile, malignancy risk, and the main clinical characteristics of the patients and associated diseases are summarized in **Table 1** [5, 16–18, 21, 22, 27, 30, 41, 50, 55–59].

Gene	Locus	Syndrome	Hormonal secretory profile	Malignancy risk	Clinical features and associated tumors
RET	10q11.2	MEN 2	Adrenergic	Low 1–5%	Frequently benign, bilateral pheochromocytomas associated with • MEN2A: Medullary thyroid carcinoma (95%) and hyperpara-thyroidism (15–30%) • MEN2B: marfanoid habitus; mucosal • Ganglioneuromas
NF1	17q11.2	NF1	Adrenergic	12%	Mostly unilateral, benign pheochromocytomas and very rare sympathetic paragangliomas, associated with: • Café- au- lait spots • Cutaneous neurofibromas • Iris hamartomas (Lisch nodules) • Optic nerve gliomas • Inguinal or axillary freckles • Sphenoid bone dysplasia or pseudoarthrosis
VHL	3p25.5	VHL	Noradrenergic	Less than 5%	Usually bilateral, benign pheochromocytomas and rare sympathetic or parasympathetic paragangliomas together with • Cerebellar and spinal hemangioblastomas • Retinal angiomas • Epididymal cystadenomas • Cysts of the broad ligament • Endolymphatic sac tumors • Clear cell renal carcinoma • Islet cell tumors of pancreas

Gene	Locus	Syndrome	Hormonal secretory profile	Malignancy risk	Clinical features and associated tumors
SDHA	5p15		Unknown	0–14%	Pheochromocytomas and paragangliomas • Leigh syndrome in homozygous patients
SDHAF2/SDH5	11q13.1 Paternal transmission	PGL2	Unknown	Unknown	Head and neck paragangliomas
SDHB	1p36.13	PGL4	Noradrenergic or dopaminergic	30–72%	Frequently malignant pheochromocytomas and sympathetic or parasympathetic head and neck paragangliomas associated with • Gastrointestinal stromal tumors • Renal cell carcinoma • Breast carcinoma • Papillary thyroid carcinoma • Neuroblastoma
SDHC	1q21	PGL3	Noradrenergic, dopaminergic or silent	Low	Mostly benign parasympathetic head and neck paragangliomas and rarely cases of pheochromocytomas and sympathetic paragangliomas
SDHD	11q23 Paternal transmission	PGL1	Noradrenergic, dopaminergic or silent	Less than 5%	Frequently multiple head and neck paragangliomas, less commonly sympathetic paragangliomas and rarely pheochromocytomas
MAX	14q23.3 Paternal transmission	–	Adrenergic or noradrenergic	25%	Frequently bilateral pheochromocytomas and paragangliomas
TMEM127	2q11.2	–	Adrenergic or noradrenergic	Low 1%	Pheochromocytomas (unilateral or bilateral), sympathetic and head and neck paragangliomas • Papillary thyroid carcinoma • Breast carcinoma

Gene	Locus	Syndrome	Hormonal secretory profile	Malignancy risk	Clinical features and associated tumors
HIF2A	2p21	Pacak-Zhuang	Noradrenergic or adrenergic	Unknown	Multiple pheochromocytomas or paragangliomas associated with: • Multiple somatostatinomas • Polycythemia
IDH	2q33.3	–	Unknown	Unknown	Carotid paragangliomas with • Glioblastoma multiforme
FH	1q43	–	Noradrenergic	Unknown/ potentially high	Pheochromocytomas associated with • Leiomyomatosis • Clear renal cell carcinoma
KIF1Bβ	1p36.2	–	Unknown	Unknown	Unilateral or bilateral Pheos, associated with • Neuroblastoma • Ganglioneuroma • Medulloblastoma • Leiomyosarcoma • Lung adenocarcinoma
PHD2/EGLN1	1q42.1	–	Unknown	Unknown	Multiple paragangliomas associated with • Erythrocytosis
H-RAS **K-RAS**	11p15 12p12	–	Adrenergic or noradrenergic	Unknown	Pheochromocytomas and paragangliomas

http://dx.doi.org/10.5772/67374

Gene	Locus	Syndrome	Hormonal secretory profile	Malignancy risk	Clinical features and associated tumors
BAP1	3p21.1	–	Unknown	Unknown	Paragangliomas associated with • Meningioma • Melanoma • Mesothelioma
ATRX	Xq21.1	–	Unknown	Unknown	Pheochromocytomas and paragangliomas
PHD1/EGLN2	19q13.2	–	Unknown	Unknown	Pheochromocytomas and paragangliomas associated with • Polycythemia
MDH2	7q11.23	–	Noradrenergic	Unknown	Multiple metastatic paragangliomas

Table 1. Genotype-phenotype correlations for pheochromocytomas and paragangliomas.

3. Guidelines for the genetic diagnosis of pheochromocytomas and paragangliomas

It is currently recognized that 30–40% of pheochromocytomas and paragangliomas are caused by the aforementioned genetic mutations, and several studies have concluded that all patients with such tumors should be genetically tested [45, 46]. Hereditary pheochromocytomas and paragangliomas are frequently multifocal, recurrent and, in particular cases, have a high risk for malignant transformation. Therefore, early diagnosis may assure more effective treatment and improved prognosis. Genetically, inherited syndromes are also commonly associated with other neoplasms, justifying the need for early diagnosis and treatment. Furthermore, the identification of a germline defect within a family can ensure early diagnosis, treatment, and better clinical outcomes for other family members. Finally, hereditary pheochromocytomas and paragangliomas should be suspected in all patients, but these cases presenting the following clinical characteristics should be investigated first: patients with clinical features of a specific syndrome, age <45 years, patients with multiple, recurrent, or malignant tumors, and also individuals with a family history or personal medical history of head and neck paragangliomas [45–47].

Management of such patients should start with a careful clinical examination including cutaneous and retinal examination followed by a genetic work-up (family history and pedigree). Advanced medical techniques such as next-generation and whole genome sequencing represent the optimal genetic strategies for discovering gene mutations [46–48]. Several studies have proposed different algorithms for genetic diagnosis in order to prioritize gene testing due to its high price and lack of availability. Patient's age and family history, together with tumor secretory profile and position are considered valuable in the determination for genetic testing. The authors propose an algorithm (**Figure 1**) for genetic testing that comprises information and clinical data from the latest medical reports [16–18, 27, 30, 41, 45–50].

Patients with a known familial disorder, syndromic lesions, or both should be tested for the appropriate gene. Specific clinical characteristics of a particular syndrome should guide the testing protocol. For example, the occurrence of MTC together with pheochromocytoma is suggestive for MEN2 (RET gene); the presence of café- au- lait spots, Lisch nodules, would indicate NF1 gene testing and the presence of hemangioblastomas significant for VHL gene testing [19–22]. In addition, the association of diseases such as GIST, renal clear cell carcinoma, breast, and thyroid carcinoma should guide the clinician to test SDH gene mutations, especially SDHB [23, 27, 28, 30].

Recent discoveries have shown that the order of tested genes in nonsyndromic, nonfamilial cases can be based on the histological evaluation, location, and biochemical phenotype of pheochromocytomas and paragangliomas. Biochemical testing is the least expensive diagnostic method, but it is often overlooked by physicians. There are several types of biochemical phenotypes:

a. The adrenergic phenotype consisting of epinephrine or metanephrine secretion orient the diagnosis first to MEN2 syndrome or NF1, then second to TMEM127, HIF2A, MAX, H-RAS, and K-RAS genes.

b. The noradrenergic phenotype, resulting in normetanephrines and norepinephrine production, is typical for pheochromocytomas within VHL disease or for SDHB-related

http://dx.doi.org/10.5772/67374

paragangliomas. However, mutations of SDHC, SDHD, MAX, HIF2A, TMEM127, FH, MDH2, K-RAS, and H-RAS genes have been reported.

c. A mixed phenotype characterized by the production of both epinephrines/metanephrines and norepinephrines/normetanephrines indicate the involvement of HIF2A, TMEM127, H-RAS, K-RAS, and MAX genes.

d. A dopaminergic biochemical phenotype should indicate first, initial SDHB and SDHD gene testing, and second, screening for SDHC gene [2, 3, 51].

e. A silent phenotype with no catecholamines/metanephrines production is associated with SDHx mutations.

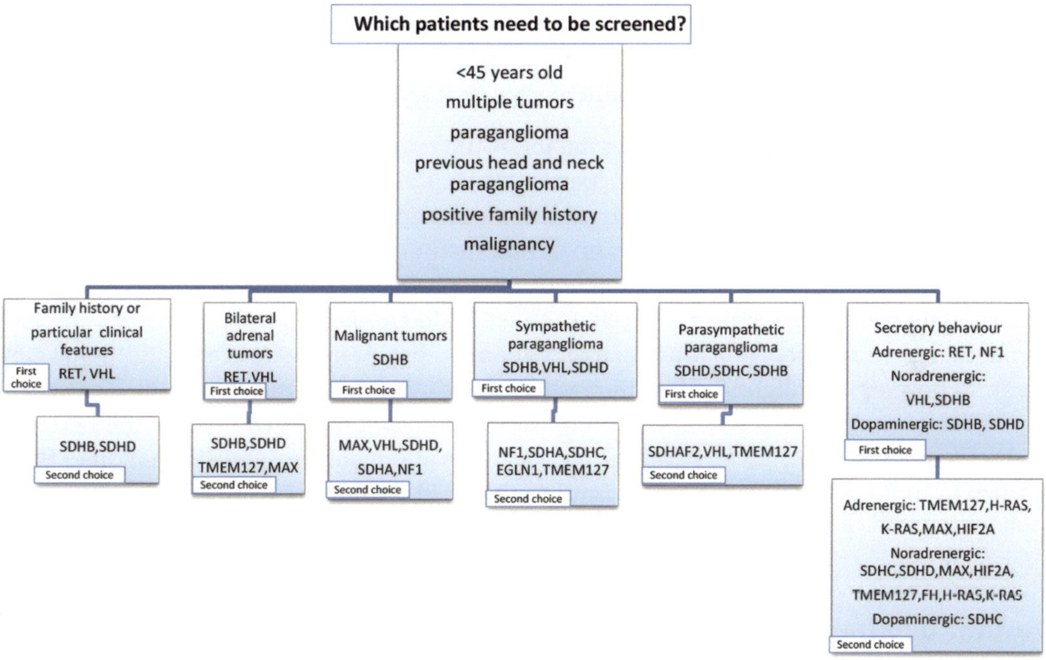

Figure 1. Genetic testing algorithm.

Bilateral pheochromocytomas are frequently described in RET and VHL gene mutations, and therefore, testing of these sites should be considered as a first step [19, 21, 41]. Afterward, if negative, mutations in SDHB, SDHD, MAX, and TMEM127 genes should be evaluated [30–33, 52, 53].

Sympathetic paragangliomas are more commonly associated with SDHB, SDHD, and VHL genes mutations; and less frequently with SDHA, SDHC, TMEM127, NF1, and EGLN1/PHD2 gene mutations [24–28, 53, 54]. Parasympathetic head and neck paragangliomas are commonly described in SDHB, SDHC, and SDHD gene mutation carriers, and rarely associated with SDHAF2, VHL, and TMEM127 gene mutations [54, 55]. Malignant pheochromocytomas and paragangliomas have been associated with germline mutations of the SDHB gene, but if negative, testing for SDHD, SDHA, VHL, MAX, and NF1 gene mutations should be considered [4, 5, 11–14, 56–59]. Moreover, paternal transmission mode of pheochromocytomas and paragangliomas corresponding to maternal imprinting leads to genetic testing toward the SDHD, SDHAF2, and MAX genes [23–25, 30, 33].

4. Conclusions

Recent progress in the better understanding of pheochromocytomas and paragangliomas have revealed 30–40% of these tumors have underlying genetic mutations. More than 21 genetic mutations involving the following genes: RET, SDHA, SDHB, SDHC, SDHD, SDHAF2, NF1, VHL, MAX, H-RAS, K-RAS, KIF1B, TMEM127, HIF2A, IDH, FH, PHD2/EGLN1, PHD1, MDH2, BAP1, and ATRX have been linked to the development of pheochromocytomas and paragangliomas. Due to cost and lack of availability of the next-generation sequencing tests used for genetic screening, it is important to classify the risks by other clinical means as well.

Recent studies recommend considering the following criteria: tumor type, position, presence of metastases, secretory profile, or any particular clinical feature. As a result, establishing a genetic testing protocol based on which physicians can guide their diagnosis and treatment is essential. The advantages of the detection of inherited mutations in cases of pheochromocytomas and paragangliomas can provide a proper diagnosis and treatment with an improved clinical outcome for the patient, as well as an early diagnosis for family members. In cases of familial pheochromocytomas and paragangliomas, distant metastases and additional cancers can develop, highlighting the importance of early diagnosis and treatment. The strong genetic determinism of pheochromocytomas and paragangliomas emphasize the need for further studies to better understand the pathogenesis and malignant transformation of these particular tumors, which may have an important role in the development of future treatment options.

Author details

Diana Loreta Păun[1, 2*] and Alexandra Mirică[1]

*Address all correspondence to: dianaloreta_paun@yahoo.com

1 C.I.Parhon, National Institute of Endocrinology, Bucharest, Romania

2 Carol Davila University of Medicine and Pharmacy, Bucharest, Romania

References

[1] DeLellis R, Lloyd R, Heitz P, Eng P. Pathology and Genetics of Tumours of Endocrine Organs (IARC WHO Classification of Tumours), IARC Press, Lyon, France, 2004.

[2] Duinen N, Corssmit EP, Jong WH, Brookman D, Kema IP, Romijn JA. Plasma levels of free metanephrines and 3-methoxytyramine indicate a higher number of biochemically active HNPGL than 24-h urinary excretion rates of catecholamines and metabolites. Eur J Endocrinol. 2013; 169:377–382.

[3] Duinen N, Steenvoorden D, Kema IP, Jansen JC, Vriends AH, Bayley JP, Smit JW, Romijn JA & Corssmit EP. Increased urinary excretion of 3-methoxytyramine in patients with head and neck paragangliomas. J Clin Endocrinol Metab. 2010; 95:209–214.

[4] Jansen JC, van den Berg R, Kuiper A, van der Mey AG, Zwinderman AH, Cornelisse CJ. Estimation of growth rate in patients with head and neck paragangliomas influences the treatment proposal. Cancer. 2000; 88:2811–2816.

[5] Gimenez-Roqueplo AP, Dahia PL & Robledo M. An update on the genetics of paraganglioma, pheochromocytoma, and associated hereditary syndromes. Horm Metab Res. 2012; 44:328–333.

[6] Chen H, Sippel RS, O'Dorisio MS, Vinik AI, Lloyd RV & Pacak K. The North American Neuroendocrine Tumor Society consensus guideline for the diagnosis and management of neuroendocrine tumors: pheochromocytoma, paraganglioma, and medullary thyroid cancer. Pancreas. 2010; 39:775–783.

[7] Kasperlik-Zaluska AA, Roslonowska E, Slowinska-Srzednicka J, et al. 1,111 patients with adrenal incidentalomas observed at a single endocrinological center: incidence of chromaffin tumors. Ann N Y Acad Sci. 2006; 1073:38–46.

[8] Scholz T, Schulz C, Klose S & Lehnert H. Diagnostic management of benign and malignant pheochromocytoma. Exp Clin Endocrinol Diabetes. 2007; 115:155–159.

[9] Thompson LD. Pheochromocytoma of the Adrenal gland Scaled Score (PASS) to separate benign from malignant neoplasms: a clinicopathologic and immunophenotypic study of 100 cases. Am J Surg Pathol. 2002; 26:551–566.

[10] Agarwal A, Mehrotra PK, Jain M, et al. Size of the tumor and pheochromocytoma of the adrenal gland scaled score (PASS): can they predict malignancy?. World J Surg. 2010; 34:3022–3028.

[11] Parenti G, Zampetti B, Rapizzi E, Ercolino T, Giache V, Mannelli M. Updated and new perspectives on diagnosis, prognosis, and therapy of malignant pheochromocytoma/paraganglioma. J Oncol. 2012; 2012:872713.

[12] Ayala-Ramirez M, Feng L, Johnson MM, et al. Clinical risk factors for malignancy and overall survival in patients with pheochromocytomas and sympathetic paragangliomas: primary tumor size and primary tumor location as prognostic indicators. J Clin Endocrinol Metab. 2011 Mar;96(3):717–725.

[13] Szalat A, Fraenkel M, Doviner V, Salmon A, Gross DJ. Malignant pheochromocytoma: predictive factors of malignancy and clinical course in 16 patients at a single tertiary medical center. Endocrine. 2011; 39:160–166.

[14] Feng F, Zhu Y, Wang X, Wu Y, Zhou W, Jin X, Zhang R, Sun F, Kasoma Z, Shen Z, Predictive factors for malignant pheochromocytoma: analysis of 136 patients. J Urol. 2011; 185(5):1583–1590.

[15] Zelinka T, Musil Z, Duskova J, et al. Metastatic pheochromocytoma: does the size and age matter?. Eur J Clin Invest. 2011; 41:1121–1128.

[16] Karasek D, Shah U, Frysak Z, Stratakis CA, Pacak K. An update on the genetics of phaeochromocytoma. J Hum Hypertens. 2012; 27:141–147.

[17] Burnichon N, Vescovo L, Amar L, Libe R, De Reynies A, et al. Integrative genomic analysis reveals somatic mutations in pheochromocytoma and paraganglioma. Hum Mol Genet. 2011; 20:3974–3985.

[18] Vicha A, Musil Z, Pacak K. Genetics of pheochromocytoma and paraganglioma syndromes: new advances and future treatment options. Curr Opin Endocrinol Diabetes Obes. 2013; 20:186–191.

[19] Bugalho MJ, Domingues R, Sobrinho L, Molecular diagnosis of multiple endocrine neoplasia Type 2. Expert Rev Mol Diagn. 2003; 3(6):769–779.

[20] Bausch B, Borozdin W, Neumann HP. European-American Pheochromocytoma Study Group. Clinical and genetic characteristics of patients with neurofibromatosis type 1 and pheochromocytoma. N Engl J Med. 2006; 354:2729–2731.

[21] Benn DE, Robinson BG. Genetic basis of phaeochromocytoma and paraganglioma. Best Pract Res Clin Endocrinol Metab. 2006; 20:435–450.

[22] Bryant J, Farmer J, Kessler LJ, Townsend RR, Nathanson KL. Pheochromocytoma: the expanding genetic differential diagnosis. J Natl Cancer Inst. 2003; 95:1196–1204.

[23] Gottlieb E, Tomlinson IPM. Mitochondrial tumour suppressors: a genetic and biochemical update. Nat Rev Cancer. 2005; 5(11):857–866.

[24] Baysal BE, Ferrell RE, Willett-Brozick JE, et al. Mutations in SDHD, a mitochondrial complex II gene, in hereditary paraganglioma. Science. 2000; 287:848–851.

[25] Hao HX, Khalimonchuk O, Schraders M, et al. SDH5, a gene required for flavination of succinate dehydrogenase, is mutated in paraganglioma. Science. 2009; 325:1139–1142

[26] Niemann S, Muller U. Mutations in SDHC cause autosomal dominant paraganglioma, type 3. Nat Genet. 2000; 26:268–270.

[27] Timmers H, Kozupa A, Eisenhofer G, et al. Clinical presentations, biochemical phenotypes, and genotype-phenotype correlations in patients with succinate dehydrogenase subunit B-associated pheochromocytomas and paragangliomas. J Clin Endocrinol Metab. 2007; 92(3):779–786.

[28] Srirangalingam U, Walker L, Khoo B, et al. Clinical manifestations of familial paraganglioma and phaeochromocytomas in succinate dehydrogenase B (SDH-B) gene mutation carriers. Clin Endocrinol. 2000; 69(4):587–596.

[29] Burnichon N, Briere JJ, Libe R, et al. SDHA is a tumor suppressor gene causing paraganglioma. Hum Mol Genet. 2010; 19:3011–3020.

[30] Timmers H, Gimenez-Roqueplo A, Mannelli M, Pacak K. Clinical aspects of SDHx-related pheochromocytoma and paraganglioma. Endocr Relat Cancer. 2009; 16(2):391–400.

[31] Yao L, Schiavi F, Cascon A, Qin Y, Inglada-Pérez L, King EE, et al. Spectrum and prevalence of FP/TMEM127 gene mutations in pheochromocytomas and paragangliomas. JAMA. 2010; 304:2611–2619.

[32] Jiang S, Dahia PLM. Minireview: the busy road to pheochromocytomas and paragangliomas has a new member, TMEM127. Endocrinology. 2011; 152:2133–2140.

[33] Burnichon N, Cascon A, Schiavi F, et al. MAX mutations cause hereditary and sporadic pheochromocytoma and paraganglioma. Clin Cancer Res. 2012; 18:2828–2837.

[34] Yang C, Sun MG, Matro J, Huynh TT, Rahimpour S, Prchal JT, Lechan R, Lonser R, Pacak K, Zhuang Z, Novel HIF2A mutations disrupt oxygen sensing, leading to polycythemia, paragangliomas, and somatostatinomas. Blood. 2013; 121(13):2563–2566.

[35] Ladroue C, Carcenac R, Leporrier M, et al. PHD2 mutation and congenital erythrocytosis with paraganglioma. N Engl J Med. 2008; 359(25):2685–2692

[36] Yeh I, Lenci R, Qin Y, et al. A germline mutation of the KIF1Bβ gene on 1p36 in a family with neural and nonneural tumors. Hum Genet. 2008; 124(3):279–285.

[37] Gaal J, Burnichon N, Korpershoek E, et al. Isocitrate dehydrogenase mutations are rare in pheochromocytomas and paragangliomas. J Clin Endocrinol Metab. 2010; 95:1274–1278.

[38] Tomlinson IPM, Alam NA, Rowan AJ, et al. Germline mutations in FH predispose to dominantly inherited uterine fibroids, skin leiomyomata and papillary renal cell cancer. Nat Genet. 2002; 30:406–410.

[39] Wadt K, Cho J, Chung JY, et al. A cryptic BAP1 splice mutation in a family with uveal and cutaneous melanoma, and paraganglioma. Pigment Cell Melanoma Res. 2012; 25:815–818.

[40] Crona J, Delgado Verdugo A, Maharjan R, et al. Somatic mutations in H-RAS in sporadic pheochromocytoma and paraganglioma identified by exome sequencing. J Clin Endocrinol Metab. 2013; 98:E1266–E1271.

[41] Crona J, Nordling M, Maharjan R, et al. Integrative genetic characterization and phenotype correlations in pheochromocytoma and paraganglioma tumours. PLoS One. 2014; 9(1): e86756.

[42] Cascon A, et al. Whole-exome sequencing identifies MDH2 as a new familial glioma gene. J Natl Cancer Inst. 2015; 107(5): djv053.

[43] Fishbein L, Khare S, et al. Whole exome sequencing identifies somatic ATRX mutations in pheochromocytomas and paragangliomas. Nat Commun. 2015; 6:6140.

[44] Yang C, Zhuang Z, et al. Germ-line PHD1 and PHD2 mutations detected in patients with pheochromocytoma/paraganglioma-polycythemia. J Mol Med (Berl). 2015; 93(1):93–104.

[45] Mannelli M, Castellano M, Schiavi F, et al. Clinically guided genetic screening in a large cohort of Italian patients with pheochromocytomas and/or functional or nonfunctional paragangliomas. J Clin Endocrinol Metab. 2009; 94(5):1541–1547.

[46] Gimenez-Roqueplo AP, Lehnert H, Mannelli M, et al. Phaeochromocytoma, new genes and screening strategies. Clin Endocrinol. 2006; 65(6):699–705.

[47] Erlic Z, Rybicki L, Pęczkowska M, et al. Clinical predictors and algorithm for the genetic diagnosis of pheochromocytoma patients. Clin Cancer Res. 2009; 15(20):6378–6385.

[48] Rattenberry E, Vialard L, Yeung A, et al. A comprehensive next generation sequencing-based genetic testing strategy to improve diagnosis of inherited pheochromocytoma and paraganglioma. J Clin Endocrinol Metab. 2013; 98:E1248–E1256.

[49] Neumann H. Pheochromocytoma. in Harrison's Principles of Internal Medicine 2011, Longo DL, Fauci AS, Kasper DL, Hauser SL, Jameson JL, and Loscalzo J, Eds., vol. 2, pp. 2962–2967, McGraw-Hill, New York, NY, USA, 18th edition.

[50] Galan SR, Kann PH. Genetics and molecular pathogenesis of pheochromocytoma and paraganglioma. Clin Endocrinol (Oxf). 2013; 78(2):165–175.

[51] Eisenhofer G, Lenders JWM, Timmers H, et al. Measurements of plasma methoxy-tyramine, normetanephrine, and metanephrine as discriminators of different hereditary forms of pheochromocytoma. Clin Chem. 2011; 57:411–420.

[52] Amar L, Bertherat J, Baudin E, Ajzenberg C, Bressac-de Paillerets B, Chabre O, et al. Genetic testing in pheochromocytoma or functional paraganglioma. J Clin Oncol. 2005; 23:8812–8818.

[53] Burnichon N, Rohmer V, Amar L, Herman P, Leboulleux S, Darrouzet V, et al. PGL.NET network. The succinate dehydrogenase genetic testing in a large prospective series of patients with paragangliomas. J Clin Endocrinol Metab. 2009; 94:2817–2827.

[54] Hensen EF, Bayley JP. Recent advances in the genetics of SDH-related paraganglioma and pheochromocytoma. Fam Cancer. 2011; 10:355–363.

[55] Welander J, Söderkvist P, Gimm O. Genetics and clinical characteristics of hereditary pheochromocytomas and paragangliomas. Endocr Relat Cancer. 2011; 18:R253–R276.

[56] Brouwers FM, Eisenhofer G, Tao JJ, Kant JA, Adams KT, Linehan WM, et al. High frequency of SDHB germline mutations in patients with malignant catecholamine-producing paragangliomas: implications for genetic testing. J Clin Endocrinol Metab. 2006; 91:4505–4509.

[57] Amar L, Baudin E, Burnichon N, Peyrard S, Silvera S, Bertherat J, et al. Succinate dehydrogenase B gene mutations predict survival in patients with malignant pheochromocytomas or paragangliomas. J Clin Endocrinol Metab. 2007; 92:3822–3828.

[58] Jochmanova I, Zelinka T, Widimsky J, Pacak K. HIF signaling pathway in pheochromocytoma and other neuroendocrine tumors. Physiol Res. 2014; 63(Suppl. 2):S251–S262.

[59] Martucci I, Pacak K. Pheochromocytoma and paraganglioma: diagnosis, genetics, management, and treatment. Curr Probl Cancer. 2014; 38(1):7–41.

Chapter 4

Rational Approach to a Patient with Suspected Primary Aldosteronism

Tomaz Kocjan

Additional information is available at the end of the chapter

http://dx.doi.org/10.5772/66965

Abstract

Primary aldosteronism (PA) is the most common form of secondary hypertension that causes higher morbidity and mortality than equally severe essential hypertension. Bilateral PA should be treated medically with spironolactone or eplerenone, the mineralocorticoid receptor antagonists (MRA), while unilateral laparoscopic adrenalectomy is recommended for unilateral disease. Surgery cures hypertension in around 40% of patients with confirmed PA and reliably demonstrated unilateral autonomous aldosterone secretion by adrenal venous sampling (AVS). Regardless of its diagnostic value, AVS has several drawbacks, in particular high cost and invasiveness. Furthermore, only a limited number of referral centers worldwide routinely carry out the procedure. On the other hand, a small number of studies that compared the effects of surgery and MRA on the incidence of cardiovascular and renal outcomes in patients with PA found no difference between the two therapeutic options. In addition, spironolactone has been recently found to be the most effective add-on drug for the treatment of resistant hypertension. Therefore, rational selection of patients with suspected PA for AVS and surgery is of utmost importance.

Keywords: adrenalectomy, adrenal venous sampling, hypertension, mineralocorticoid receptor antagonists, primary aldosteronism

1. Introduction

Primary aldosteronism (PA) is a group of disorders in which aldosterone production is inappropriately high for sodium status, relatively autonomous and nonsuppressible by sodium loading. Such inappropriate production of aldosterone causes hypertension, sodium retention, suppression of plasma renin, and increased potassium excretion [1]. Once thought to be rare, PA is now considered the most common form of secondary hypertension with an estimated prevalence of 4.3% in primary care and of 9.5% among referred hypertensive patients [2]. Accumulated experimental and clinical evidence clearly shows that prolonged exposure to elevated aldosterone levels causes excess cardiovascular and renal damage which is partly independent of blood pressure (BP) levels [3]. Consequently, this endocrine condition is far from being benign, and patients with PA appear to have higher rates of cardiac arrhythmia, coronary heart disease, heart failure, stroke, proteinuria, and renal impairment compared to matched patients with essential hypertension (EH) [4–6]. Their cardiovascular mortality might be also increased [7]. Targeted treatment of PA is possible and is of obvious benefit to affected patients.

The Endocrine Society now explicitly recognizes PA as a major public health issue and recommends extensive screening for this disorder using the plasma aldosterone/renin ratio (ARR) in high-risk populations, including patients with sustained BP more than 150/100 mm Hg, resistant hypertension, spontaneous or diuretic-induced hypokalemia, adrenal incidentaloma, or sleep apnea. Most patients with a positive ARR should undergo one or more confirmatory tests to definitively confirm or exclude the diagnosis. Then lateralization of the source of the excessive aldosterone secretion is critical to guide the management of confirmed PA because unilateral adrenalectomy in patients with unilateral disease results in the normalization of hypokalemia; hypertension is also improved or even cured. In bilateral PA medical therapy with spironolactone or other mineralocorticoid receptor antagonists (MRA) is the treatment of choice. Unilateral disease may also be treated medically if the patient declines or is not a candidate for surgery. The first step in subtype classification is adrenal computed tomography (CT). Finally, all but few surgical candidates need cumbersome adrenal venous sampling (AVS) to reliably distinguish between unilateral and bilateral adrenal disease and to decide for optimal treatment [1].

These guidelines place a high value on avoiding the risk associated with missing a diagnosis of unilateral PA and thus the opportunity of possibly curative intervention by unilateral adrenalectomy and a lower value on avoiding the risks of exposing patients with bilateral PA (who are candidates for medical treatment) to additional diagnostic testing. As the global burden of PA seems to be very high and the recommended diagnostic procedures are complex and costly, consistent translation of the guidelines into clinical practice might not be possible even in the most affluent healthcare systems. Hence, rational approach to a patient with suspected PA seems the only option, and it will be briefly reviewed here. Several clinical situations will be presented, in order to show the different ways of medical decision-making in using the guidelines and to help the clinicians to apply these guidelines to their patients with suspected or confirmed PA.

2. Patients with suspected PA

When resources are limited, the clinician might not be able to measure plasma aldosterone concentration (PAC) and renin to determine ARR. Such patients should be treated with an MRA if they have reasonable renal function because PA is very common [2]. Moreover, there is ample, published supportive data that spironolactone is an excellent antihypertensive agent in patients with hypertension and without PA [8, 9]. Spironolactone has even been recently found to be the most effective add-on drug for the treatment of resistant hypertension [10]. Therefore, some experts propose inclusion of a low-dose MRA (spironolactone 12.5/25 mg daily or equivalent doses of another antagonist) as part of first-line therapy for all hypertensive subjects [11].

The Endocrine Society now similarly recommends medical treatment including an MRA, if an ARR-positive patient is unwilling or unable to undergo further investigations [1]. Older patients with multiple medical comorbidities who are at high surgical risk and those with short life expectancy should be included in this group [12]. Pure aldosterone-secreting adrenocortical carcinomas are exceptionally uncommon [13]; however, some form of adrenal imaging might be considered for these patients, except in cases with long-standing and mild (e.g., normokalemic) disease.

Notably, MRA, amiloride, triamterene, and potassium-wasting diuretics should be withdrawn for at least 4 weeks before ARR testing. A washout of all interfering antihypertensive medications such as angiotensin-converting enzyme inhibitors, angiotensin receptor blockers, dihydropyridine calcium channel antagonists, and beta-adrenergic blockers is feasible in patients with mild hypertension but is potentially problematic in others and is often not required if the results of ARR on the above agents are clearly diagnostic. If all potentially problematic agents cannot be safely withdrawn, an ARR should be performed and the results considered in the light of the potential confounding factors [1]. In case of very low renin levels, care should be taken to avoid overinflating ARR. Only a certain minimum value of renin can be included in the ratio. This value is often fixed at 0.2 ng/ml/h for plasma renin activity (PRA) and at 0.36 ng/ml for direct renin activity (DRA). Elderly patients and individuals of African origin usually have low renin values, and the precautions described are vital in such cases [14].

3. Patients with confirmed PA

Spontaneous hypokalemia, plasma renin below detection levels, and PAC > 20 ng/dL (>550 pmol/L) may be sufficient for the diagnosis of PA [1]. For patients without these laboratory characteristics who are undergoing confirmatory testing without MRA and thiazide diuretics, additional extensive medication switching is not always needed, because it appears that more severely excessive aldosterone overproduction (e.g., post-saline infusion test (SIT) PAC ≥ 8.6 ng/dL (>240 pmol/L)) may not be effectively suppressed by less interfering chronic antihypertensive drugs. When PA is less severe, reproducibility of confirmatory tests performed without recommended drug withdrawal is much less than optimal [15].

Patients with confirmed PA and excluded adrenocortical carcinoma by CT should not be coerced into considering AVS and surgery if they prefer not to undergo the procedures, given that there is reasonable evidence to suggest that lifelong treatment with MRA is a valid alternative to surgery. Treatment choice should, therefore, be primarily driven by the preferences of the well-informed patient. Candidates for surgery should be told that the presence of an adrenal adenoma poses no risk in terms of cancer [12]. In patients with an onset of confirmed PA earlier than 20 years of age and in those who have a family history of PA or stroke at a young age (<40 years), genetic testing for familial hyperaldosteronism type 1 (FH-I) [glucocorticoid remediable aldosteronism (GRA)] is suggested. When confirmed, FH-I should be always treated medically [1].

3.1. Medical therapy vs. surgery

In the absence of RCTs comparing surgical and medical treatment of PA may prove difficult, as a recent systematic review found. The existing studies were all carried out in a limited number of centers and were usually dealing with relatively small number of patients. Their main aim was to compare patients with PA and those with EH, but they failed to predefine medical treatment for target BP and dose or type of medication. When surgery was found the superior approach in those studies over the medical treatment of patients, it was often with groups that received no MRA or low doses of it (in some cases treatment was not reported). Furthermore, two different forms of PA, the unilateral disease and the bilateral disease, that may not be fully comparable were treated as a single one in the majority of the studies, since surgical procedures were mostly performed on patients with the former type of PA and medical treatment was delivered predominantly to those with the latter form [16]. This limits the usefulness of the results obtained, since it must be noted that patients with bilateral PA are in general less responsive to monotherapy with MRA than those with unilateral PA [17]. Comparisons between surgically and medically treated patients with PA should, therefore, be interpreted with caution [16].

The effects on improvement of BP and hypokalemia were similar in surgically and medically treated patients in six studies, and surgery was reported to be superior in another six studies [16]. Of note, in German Conn's registry, the observed all-cause mortality following adrenalectomy was reduced compared with medical treatment [7]. However, several outcome variables in PA with regard to end-organ damage appear to improve to a comparable level after medical and surgical treatment. A meta-analysis of long-term studies which included 355 patients with PA and median follow-up of 4 years showed that reduction of left ventricular mass was not different after adrenalectomy or medical treatment with MRA [18]. Furthermore, when comparing the incidence of combined cardio- and cerebrovascular events comprising myocardial infarction, stroke, any type of revascularization procedure, and sustained arrhythmias in treated patients with PA and matched controls with EH, the benefits of PA treatment were similar for specific drugs and surgery [5, 19]. Spironolactone, when uptitrated as needed and tolerated, is as effective as surgery in correcting the relative glomerular hyperfiltration and microalbuminuria of patients with PA [12]. Comparable improvement in sensitivity to insulin and glucose metabolism in surgically and medically treated PA was also reported [20]. No significant difference in prevalence of depression and anxiety was found 5.4 years after initiation of MRA treatment or 4.3 years after unilateral adrenalectomy in patients with PA [21]. Remission of bilateral PA may occur in some patients after long-term MRA treatment [22] and exceptionally also in unilateral disease [23].

On the other hand, patients treated medically need more antihypertensive drugs and require a longer follow-up and more clinical visits at specialized referral centers than those treated surgically [24]. Quality of life seems to be worse in medically treated patients with PA and improves more slowly and to a lesser degree than with surgical treatment [25]. Side effects are common in patients receiving treatment with MRA, especially spironolactone, contributing to increased healthcare consumption and increased risk of noncompliance [16]. Consequently, at least in terms of ongoing antihypertensive medication requirements and quality of life, clinical responses to unilateral adrenalectomy in patients with unilateral PA are superior to those in patients with bilateral PA treated medically. Therefore, unilateral disease in appropriately selected patients is generally recommended to be treated surgically [26]. Adrenalectomy for PA is also less expensive than long-term medical treatment for patients with PA with a life expectancy of more than 25 years, performing AVS in all patients and adrenalectomy in those displaying lateralization than not carrying out AVS and providing lifelong drug treatment for all patients [27].

3.2. Selection of patients for AVS and surgery

Laparoscopic adrenalectomy, using transperitoneal or retroperitoneal approaches, is the preferred therapeutic strategy for unilateral PA [28]. It has a morbidity of 5–14%, a mortality below 1%, and a mean hospital stay around 3 days. Adrenalectomy generally results in the normalization of aldosterone secretion and serum potassium (96–100%); however, patients should be warned that hypertension is not always cured [29]. Based on 2482 patients from 16 studies, BP was normalized in a mean of 42% (range 20–72%) of patients [16]. Of note, older studies with a "cure" rate as high as 56–77% used the cure threshold of BP < 160/95 mm Hg, which is clearly still in the hypertensive range [1].

3.2.1. Predictors of cure or persistent hypertension

Whether hypertension can be successfully cured or whether it is likely to persist can be inferred from predictors that have been extensively studied. At least one multivariate analysis found the following statistically significant predictors of hypertension persistence after adrenalectomy in patients with unilateral PA: advanced age, male gender, longer hypertension duration, higher BMI, more drug classes, higher preoperative BP, higher 24 h urinary aldosterone/active renin ratio, lower estimated GFR, higher serum potassium concentrations, or evidence of arteriolosclerosis [29]. Recently, higher renal resistive index calculated by Doppler ultrasonography has been also reported to predict worse postoperative BP outcome in PA [30]. On the other hand, a positive predictive factor for cure is histologically verified aldosterone-producing adenoma [16], especially if harboring somatic KCNJ5 (inwardly rectifying potassium channel, subfamily J, member 5 gene) mutations [31]. Recently, a study based on German Conn's registry found out that PA patients with post-SIT PAC > 10 ng/dL (>280 pmol/L) showed a better outcome after adrenalectomy regarding blood pressure, potassium normalization, and reduction in the number of antihypertensive drugs. On the other hand, low post-SIT PAC levels of 5–10 ng/dL (140–280 pmol/L) were an indicator of less successful outcome, so the authors suggested that post-SIT PAC is a predictor for the remission probability of PA post adrenalectomy [32]. Interestingly, diagnosis of unilateral PA confirmed by AVS was never found to be a predictor of good outcome after surgery, and patients with a higher lateralization index on AVS do not have a better outcome [29]. Contralateral suppression on AVS correlated with good BP and biochemical outcomes from surgery in some [33, 34], but not in all studies [35].

Few prediction models have been developed to help clinicians to objectively inform patients of likely clinical outcomes before surgical intervention. The aldosteronoma resolution score (ARS) was composed of four readily available clinical predictors (two or fewer antihypertensive medications, body mass index ≤ 25 kg/m^2, duration of hypertension ≤ 6 years, and female sex) to identify individuals at low or high likelihood of complete resolution of hypertension. However, even if none of these features were present in an individual patient, he still had a 25% probability of being completely cured by an adrenalectomy in the validation cohort [36]. A better option to predict BP cure after adrenalectomy might present a novel nomogram that has been recently developed in Japan. The included factors are the duration of hypertension, number of antihypertensive drug classes used, and age and sex for an individual patient [37]. When selecting patients for surgery, one should not attach excessive importance to these hypertension cure predictors. Namely, several of the studies conducted could not ascertain the link between these predictors and the eventual cure of the hypertension. In addition, some studies suffered from small sample sizes used in their multivariate analysis approach [29]. Factors predictive of the persistence of hypertension after adrenalectomy should not, therefore, be used as exclusive arguments for or against surgery in individual cases.

The most common reasons for persistently increased BP after adrenalectomy are coexistent EH and older age and/or longer duration of hypertension [1]. A significant number of patients who are not cured by adrenalectomy for PA will still benefit from surgery. Even if hypertension persists, the patient will experience a significant decrease in BP and/or treatment requirements. Adrenalectomy usually produces a large decrease in systolic BP (typically −25 to −40 mm Hg) and in the number of antihypertensive medications prescribed (typically −1 to −2 drug classes). Additionally, the focus on hypertension cure obscures the likely cure of hypokalemia and the normalization of aldosterone secretion which probably has BP-independent benefits [29].

3.2.2. *Subtype diagnosis*

Subtype diagnosis is required only if surgery is being considered. Adrenal venous sampling (AVS) is currently regarded as the only reliable method to distinguish bilateral from unilateral PA [38]. In order to avoid an unnecessary or an inappropriate adrenalectomy, in principle, AVS should be performed in all patients with PA who want to pursue surgical cure. AVS is preceded by CT not only to exclude large masses that may represent adrenocortical carcinoma (**Figure 1**) but also to assist the interventional radiologist (and surgeon) where anatomically appropriate [1].

Generally, adrenal CT is not accurate in distinguishing between unilateral and bilateral disease and might have misdiagnosed the type of PA in 37.8% of patients when AVS was used as the criterion standard test for diagnosing laterality of aldosterone secretion (**Figure 2**) [38].

Morphology does not predict biochemical function, and many aldosteronomas are very small with up to 42% of them being <6 mm in diameter (**Figure 3**) [39].

http://dx.doi.org/10.5772/66965

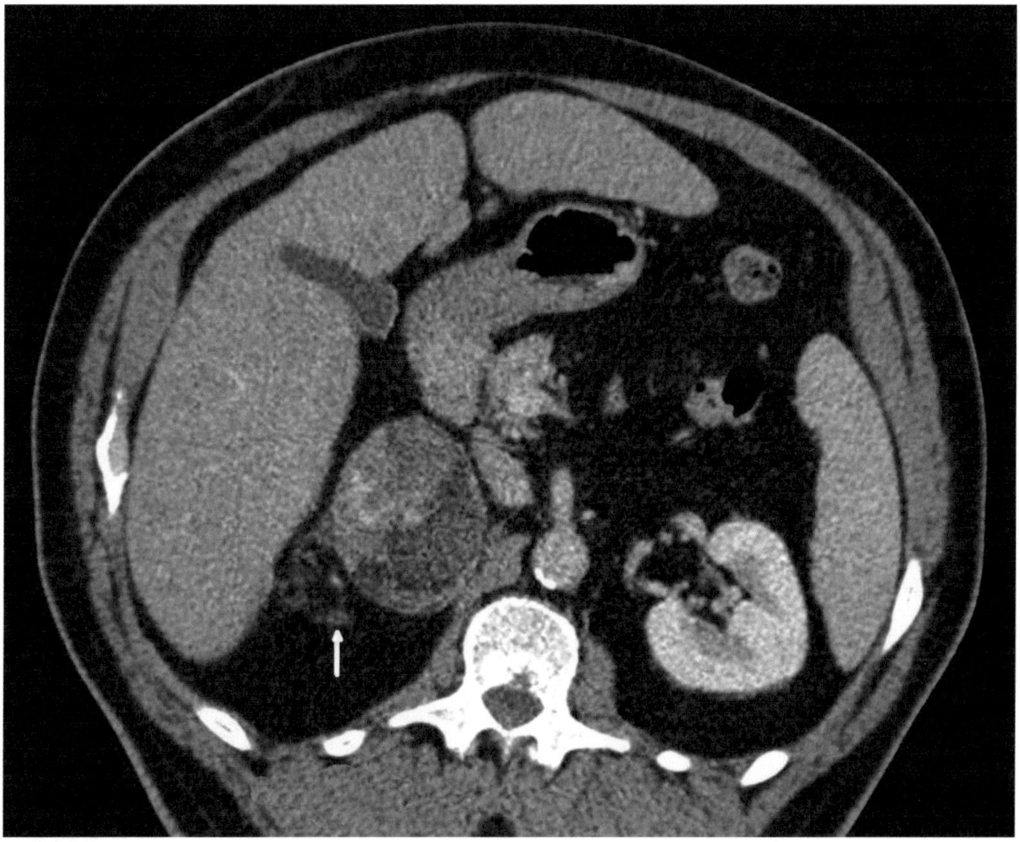

Figure 1. Adrenocortical carcinoma with mineralocorticoid activity in right adrenal gland showing typical heterogeneous appearance and local invasion (arrow) (CT scan).

However, a recent, rigorously conducted randomized controlled trial that compared the outcome of CT-based management with AVS-based management for 200 patients with PA found no difference between the groups with regard to the intensity of antihypertensive drug treatment, mean blood pressure, the proportion of patients reaching target blood pressure (<135/85 mm Hg), quality of life, or adverse events after 1 year. Moreover, there was no difference in the frequency of adrenalectomy and no statistically significant difference in biochemical failure in operated patients (11% in the AVS group vs. 20% in the CT group; $p = 0.25$) [40]. The outcome of this study is unexpected and challenges current guidelines. It is, however, important to consider that more than 70% of patients with PA present with normokalemia. This is a patient group not covered by the trial, and caution should be used in generalizing these findings [41]. In addition, when considering persistent vs. resolved PA, a nonsignificant trend in favor of AVS was found that might become statistically significant in a larger cohort [40].

Regardless of its diagnostic value, AVS has several drawbacks, in particular the lack of a standardized procedure, variable handling of cutoffs, high cost, and invasiveness. It has a

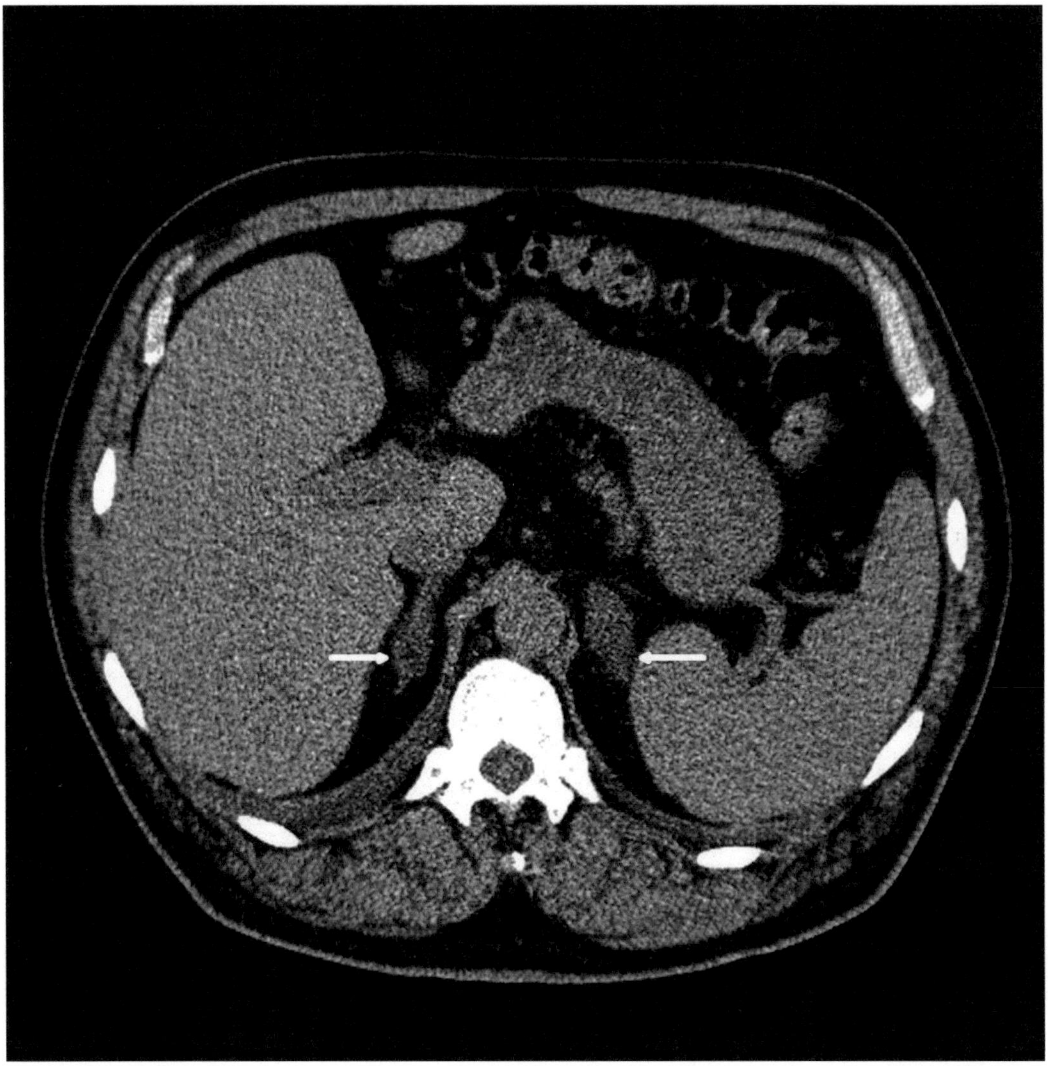

Figure 2. Bilaterally enlarged adrenal glands with aldosterone-producing adenoma (20 mm) on the right and hormonally inactive incidentaloma (30 mm) on the left (arrows) (CT scan).

reputation as a technically difficult procedure with the average success rate for cannulating the right adrenal vein of only 74% [42]. The addition of rapid intra-procedural measurement of adrenal vein cortisol concentrations is useful in centers with low success rates [43], and accuracy of catheter placement can be also improved with C-arm CT [44]. With experience the success rate can be improved to 90–96% [45]. The risk of adrenal hemorrhage can be minimized by employing a radiologist skilled in the technique, avoiding adrenal venography and limiting the use of contrast to the smallest amounts necessary to assess the catheter tip position. At centers with experienced AVS radiologists, the complication rate is 2.5% or lower [46]. More recent studies, report, however, a substantially lower rate of complications

http://dx.doi.org/10.5772/66965

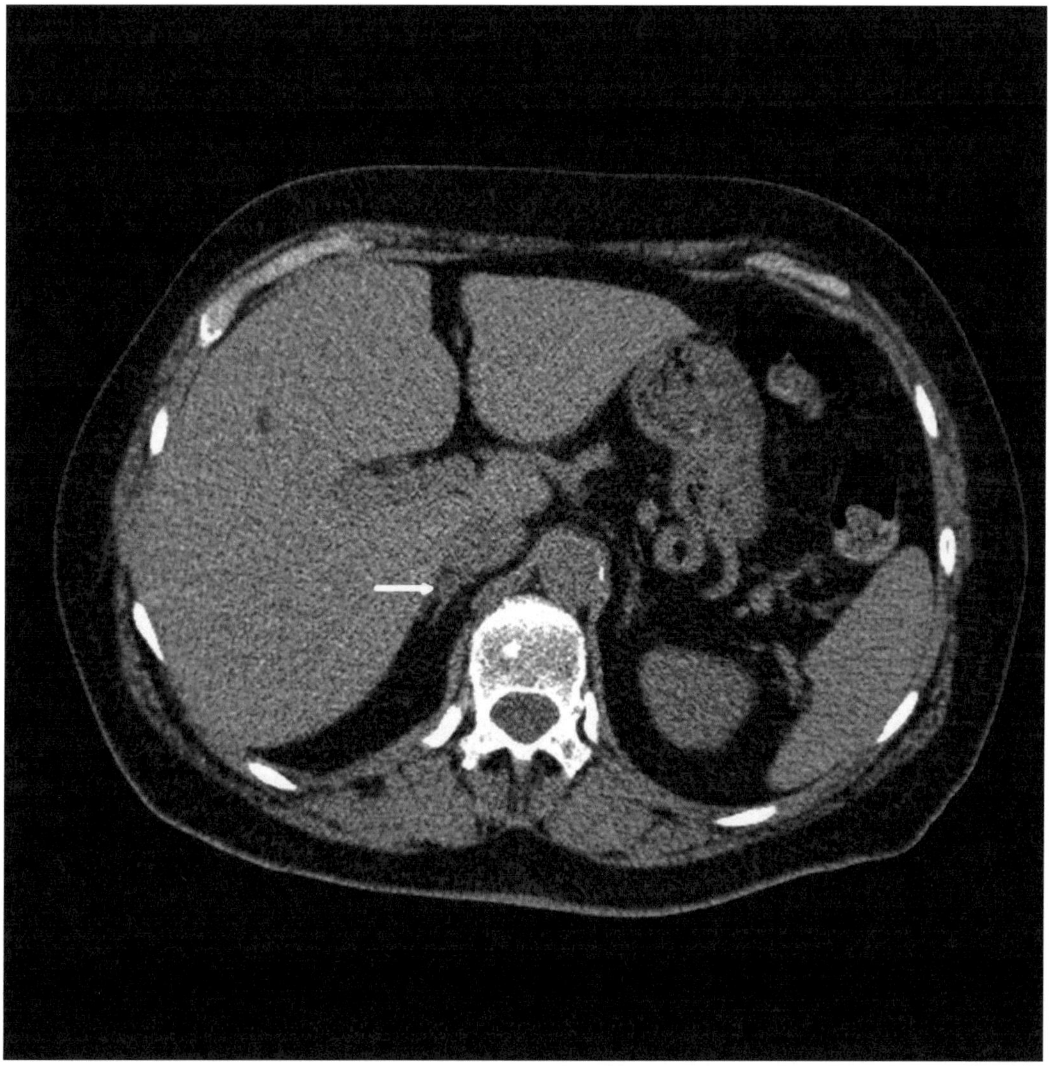

Figure 3. Tiny aldosterone producing adenoma (6 mm) in right adrenal gland (arrow) (CT scan).

of between 0.2 and 0.9%. Only a limited number of referral centers worldwide routinely carry out the procedure (**Figure 4**).

The Adrenal Vein Sampling International Study (AVIS) which explored AVS practice in 20 centers from Asia, Australia, the USA, and Europe confirmed that AVS was under-utilized with marked variation in techniques and interpretation of results and therefore highlighted a clear need for definitive guidelines on the use and interpretation of AVS in identifying unilateral aldosterone excess [47]. Importantly, different sets of criteria used to interpret AVS in different institutions translate into heterogeneous classifications and hence management decisions, for patients with PA [48]. Recently, many of these issues have been addressed by several opinion papers [26, 49]. An expert consensus statement

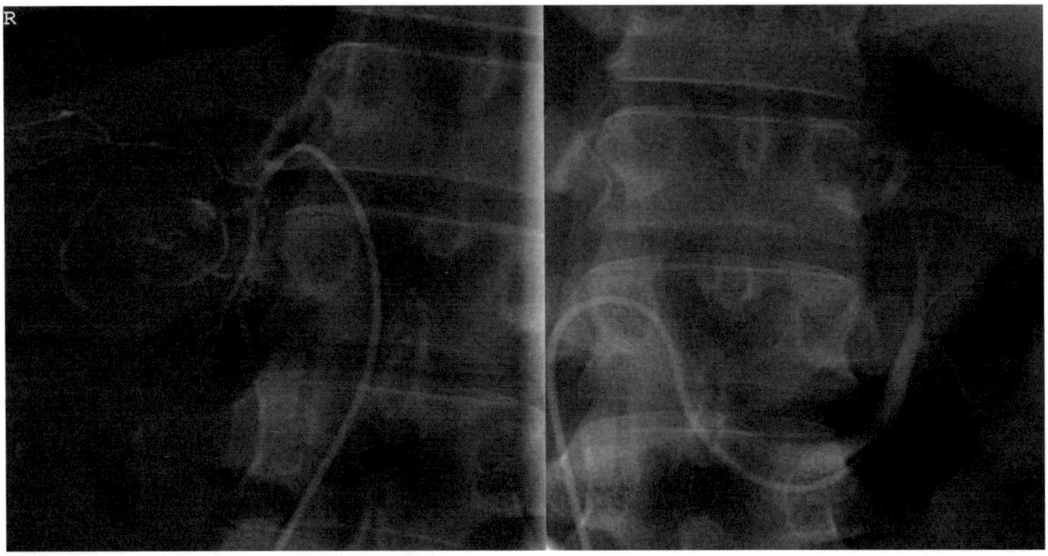

Figure 4. Adrenal venous sampling (AVS) showing right (R) and left adrenal veins.

was also reached on a number of key issues, including the preparation of the patients for the AVS, the procedure for its optimal performance, and the interpretation of its results for diagnostic purposes even in the most challenging cases [50].

Still, the most important prerequisite for overall clinical success is the selective use of AVS that should be based on patient preferences, patient age, clinical comorbidities, and the clinical probability of finding unilateral PA (**Table 1**) [45].

Most appropriate candidates for AVS are patients who desire surgery and are considered to have a high probability of unilateral PA. They have severe hypertension; higher plasma (>25 ng/dL (694 pmol/L)), and urinary (>30 μg/24 h (83 nmol/d)) levels of aldosterone; are younger (<50 years old); and have more frequent hypokalemia than those with bilateral PA [42]. For example, in a large prospective study of the prevalence of PA in 1125 hypertensive patients, spontaneous hypokalemia <3.5 mmol/L was found in only 17% of patients with bilateral PA compared to about one-half of patients with unilateral disease [51]. In another smaller study, hypokalemia (<3.6 mmol/L) was present in 74.2% of patients with unilateral PA and in 30.8% of patients with bilateral PA [52]. However, these factors are not absolute predictors of unilateral vs. bilateral adrenal disease [42].

SIT is probably the most widely used diagnostic confirmatory test for PA due to feasibility, low cost, and good compliance [1]. It is a reliable alternative to the more expensive and complex fludrocortisone suppression test [53]. There is also some evidence to support its significance for distinguishing unilateral from bilateral disease. Traditionally, it was assumed that aldosterone secretion in patients with unilateral PA appears to be relatively autonomous in response to sodium loading. On the other hand, the ability to influence aldosterone secretion was assumed to be less affected in patients with bilateral PA. Through a working, though abnormal feedback mechanism, they presumably responded

No AVS → adrenalectomy	AVS → adrenalectomy when proven unilateral PA	No AVS → medical treatment
Adrenal tumor on CT with malignant features (e.g., possible adrenocortical carcinoma) [1]	Patient preference for surgical treatment	Patient preference for medical treatment
Age < 35 years with severe PA and an unilateral adrenal macroadenoma with normal contralateral gland [1, 70]	High clinical probability of unilateral PA (e.g., severe hypertension, hypokalemia, higher basal, or post-SIT PAC, age < 50 years) [32, 42]	Patient not suitable for surgery (e.g., older age and/or multiple comorbidities)
	Positive clinical prediction score for unilateral PA [63, 67]	Positive clinical prediction criterion for bilateral PA [68]
	Persistent hypertension less likely [12, 16, 29, 36, 37]	Persistent hypertension more likely [12, 16, 29, 36, 37]
	Higher peripheral plasma 18-oxocortisol [59]	Positive genetic testing for FH-I [1]

Note: PAC, plasma aldosterone concentration; SIT, saline infusion test; FH-I, familial hyperaldosteronism type I.

Table 1. Selective use of adrenal venous sampling (AVS) in primary aldosteronism (PA).

to progressive sodium loading with decreased levels of aldosterone secretion [54]. In fact, when compared to patients with unilateral PA, such patients showed a greater level of reduction of aldosterone after SIT in a study that comprised 100 hypertensive subjects [53]. By contrast, in the PAPY study, no such differences of post-SIT aldosterone cutoffs were detected [55]. However, recent data from German Conn's registry found out that PA patients with post-SIT PAC > 10 ng/dL (>280 pmol/L) had more often unilateral disease with larger aldosteronomas and more severe clinical manifestations, while low post-SIT PAC levels of 5–10 ng/dL (140–280 pmol/L) were an indicator of more frequent bilateral disease [32]. Similarly, PAC after shortened SIT at 2 h was significantly higher in patients with unilateral PA than in those with bilateral PA; however, receiver-operated characteristic (ROC) curve analyses did not yield 100% specificity and sensitivity [56]. Apparently, post-SIT PAC levels provide additional useful information for the subtype classification, but cannot replace AVS as a reference test.

As unilateral disease is reported to be generally more sensitive to ACTH than bilateral PA, several groups explored significance of adrenocorticotropin stimulation test with or without dexamethasone suppression in determining the subtype of PA. PAC level after ACTH stimulation was effective for the diagnosis of unilateral PA. The diagnostic accuracy was around 80–90%, so this test might be used to select patients who have high probability of unilateral disease and definitely require AVS [57, 58].

Apparently, measurement of peripheral plasma 18-oxocortisol could contribute to the clinical determination between unilateral and bilateral PA. The degree of separation between the two subtypes in the study was considerable, with less than 40% of patients not able to be allocated to one or the other [59]. However, until these data are reproduced elsewhere, this surrogate may guide the clinician in selecting patients for AVS but should not be used to direct surgical management [1].

Another approach might be the preselection of patients by mass spectrometry-based peripheral venous steroid profiling for subtyping of PA, on the basis of a report showing that correct classification of 80% of cases of unilateral vs. bilateral PA was possible by the use of a combination of steroids in peripheral plasma [60]. Combining imaging information with steroid profiles might become a future strategy to spare patients who are likely to have bilateral disease from invasive and costly procedures and to select patients with a high likelihood of having unilateral PA for direct surgery or AVS [41].

Contrary to the increased PAC sensitivity to small changes in angiotensin II concentrations, induced by standing upright, which was observed in patients with bilateral PA, no such enhancement was found in those with unilateral PA where PAC displayed diurnal variation. This finding served as a basis for posture simulation test [1]. Unfortunately, some aldosteronomas are also sensitive to angiotensin II, and some patients with bilateral PA have diurnal variations in aldosterone secretion, so this test is generally not useful for subtype diagnosis [52]. It may probably serve only an ancillary role if positive for unilateral PA in those patients for whom AVS was unsuccessful and CT shows a unilateral adrenal mass [1].

3.3. Alternatives to AVS

There is a persistent, ongoing search for reliable alternative methods to recognize unilateral PA and to identify suitable candidates for adrenalectomy without AVS but with very limited success.

3.3.1. Nuclear imaging

(6β-131 I) Iodomethyl-19-norcholesterol (NP-59) scintigraphy, performed with dexamethasone suppression, has the theoretical advantage of correlating function with anatomical abnormalities. However, the sensitivity of this test is poor in adenomas smaller than 1.5 cm in diameter, so it rarely plays a role in subtype evaluation [1]. (11)C-Metomidate PET-CT has been presented as a sensitive and specific noninvasive alternative to AVS in the management of PA (**Figure 5**) [61].

These data have not been confirmed by subsequent studies. Moreover, metomidate has low selectivity for aldosterone synthase (CYP11B2) over 11β-hydroxylase (CYP11B1), which affects its specificity for visualization of aldosterone-producing adenomas [41]. A new preclinical study reported on (18)F-CDP2230, a specific aldosterone synthase tracer with a high selectivity for imaging zona glomerulosa that might become a promising tool for detecting unilateral subtypes of PA in the future [62].

3.3.2. Clinical prediction scores

Identification of unilateral PA with the help of a clinical prediction score has been proposed. According to the original study, the score exhibits 100% specificity for unilateral disease if either serum potassium concentration is lower than 3.5 mmol/L or an estimated glomerular filtration rate equals or exceeds 100 mL/min/1.73 m^2, while at the same time, a unilateral adenoma of at least 8 mm in size has to be identifiable on a CT scan. Authors suggested that 30% percent of the included patients would have been appropriately diagnosed as lateralized

http://dx.doi.org/10.5772/66965

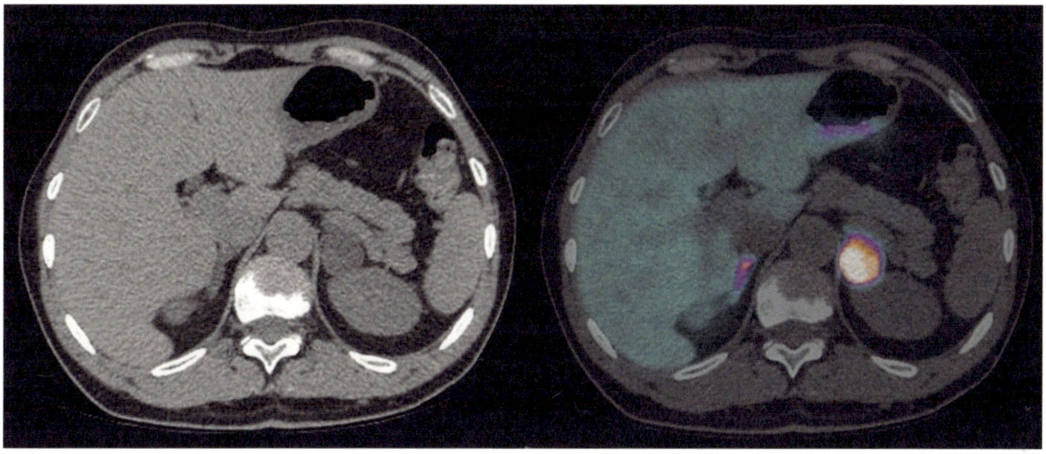

Figure 5. A relatively large nodule (30 mm) in left adrenal gland (CT scan) with high tracer uptake on (11)C-metomidate PET-CT scan identified as aldosterone-producing adenoma.

based on these criteria without AVS [63]. But when later validated against international databases in three separate studies, the proposed score's specificity was seen to drop to between 80 and 88.5%, making its reliability questionable [64–66]. A different recently developed subtype prediction score incorporated PAC, serum potassium, and ARR in a post-captopril challenge test but failed to achieve 100% specificity for unilateral PA even within the test group [67].

Therefore, most previous attempts to predict unilateral PA without AVS ultimately failed and could have led to wrong decisions for adrenalectomy. It might be more reasonable to avoid AVS only when this would not permanently influence clinical management. Patients with bilateral disease have the most prevalent form of PA and are usually treated medically, so we recently suggested that identification of patients with bilateral PA might be the right approach to decide for or against AVS. We conducted a retrospective diagnostic study at our center, in order to find variables associated with nonlateralized AVS. Combining the identified predictors, namely, serum potassium ≥ 3.5 mmol/L, post-SIT aldosterone < 18 ng/dL (<500 pmol/L), and either no or bilateral tumor found on CT imaging into a single criterion for predicting nonlateralized AVS seemed a better approach than establishing another score with uncertain validity. In patients with bilateral PA, the sensitivity of the combined criterion was determined to be modest (28.2%), but the approach yielded perfect specificity and therefore a positive predictive value of 100% [68]. If this rule is validated on an independent sample, patients with all three incorporated variables that are readily available and intuitively associated with bilateral PA by themselves [32, 42, 52] could avoid AVS and immediately start with medical treatment. Last but not least, it is important to emphasize that even if the proposed criterion proved wrong in some cases, its use would still be perfectly safe for the patient, because it does not attempt to predict unilateral PA as some other authors unsuccessfully did [63, 67]. While adrenalectomy is not without risk and its effects cannot be reversed, medical treatment could be stopped anytime, and the patient could proceed to AVS and surgery if clinically plausible. Although potentially optimal, surgery is not mandatory for PA caused by unilateral disease, and the option of medical treatment with MRA should be discussed with all patients [12].

3.4. Patients with PA proceeding to surgery without AVS

It is not possible to avoid AVS in most individuals with PA who are candidates for surgery [1]. There are few exceptions to this rule. In the past, it was proposed by the Mayo Clinic group that in patients younger than 40 years with severe PA, marked spontaneous hypokalemia, and a clearly visible unilateral adrenal cortical macroadenoma (>1 cm and <2 cm in diameter) in imaging, AVS is not necessary [69]. Unfortunately, more recent data from the same authors showed some false positives even in this age group, and CT imaging was 100% concordant with AVS only in a small subgroup of patients with PA, who were younger than 35 years of age [70]. Similarly, in German Conn's registry, it was not possible to rely on imaging alone after classification of patients with an age of 40 years or younger. On the other hand, the clinical prediction score for unilateral PA [63] achieved a specificity of 100% when used in the same cohort [64].

4. Conclusion

A careful selection of patients for AVS is possible and should be ideally undertaken in all patients with PA who pursue the surgical management except in infrequent younger patients with Conn's adenoma who could probably proceed directly to unilateral adrenalectomy. Naturally, AVS is not needed in some patients who prefer medical therapy over an adrenalectomy and in those who are not suitable for surgery due to comorbidities or age. If validated on an independent sample, our simple clinical prediction criterion could accurately determine a subset of patients with bilateral PA who should avoid unnecessary AVS and immediately commence with medical treatment. In addition, a careful identification of prospectively evaluated factors associated with long-term BP control after adrenalectomy should guide preoperative individual patient counseling and ultimate decision for or against AVS and surgery.

Author details

Tomaz Kocjan

Address all correspondence to: tomaz.kocjan@kclj.si

Department of Endocrinology, Diabetes and Metabolic Diseases, University Medical Centre Ljubljana, Ljubljana, Slovenia

References

[1] Funder JW, Carey RM, Mantero F, Murad MH, Reincke M, Shibata H, et al. The management of primary aldosteronism: case detection, diagnosis, and treatment: an endocrine society clinical practice guideline. J Clin Endocrinol Metab. 2016;101:1889-916.

[2] Hannemann A, Wallaschofski H. Prevalence of primary aldosteronism in patient's cohorts and in population-based studies--a review of the current literature. Horm Metab Res. 2012;44:157-62.

[3] Rossi G-P, Sechi LA, Giacchetti G, Ronconi V, Strazzullo P, Funder JW. Primary aldosteronism: cardiovascular, renal and metabolic implications. Trends Endocrinol Metab TEM. 2008;19:88-90.

[4] Savard S, Amar L, Plouin P-F, Steichen O. Cardiovascular complications associated with primary aldosteronism: a controlled cross-sectional study. Hypertension. 2013;62:331-6.

[5] Mulatero P, Monticone S, Bertello C, Viola A, Tizzani D, Iannaccone A, et al. Long-term cardio- and cerebrovascular events in patients with primary aldosteronism. J Clin Endocrinol Metab. 2013;98:4826-33.

[6] Reincke M, Rump LC, Quinkler M, Hahner S, Diederich S, Lorenz R, et al. Risk factors associated with a low glomerular filtration rate in primary aldosteronism. J Clin Endocrinol Metab. 2009;94:869-75.

[7] Reincke M, Fischer E, Gerum S, Merkle K, Schulz S, Pallauf A, et al. Observational study mortality in treated primary aldosteronism: the German Conn's registry. Hypertens. 2012;60:618-24.

[8] Ouzan J, Pérault C, Lincoff AM, Carré E, Mertes M. The role of spironolactone in the treatment of patients with refractory hypertension. Am J Hypertens. 2002;15:333-9.

[9] Eide IK, Torjesen PA, Drolsum A, Babovic A, Lilledahl NP. Low-renin status in therapy-resistant hypertension: a clue to efficient treatment. J Hypertens. 2004;22:2217-26.

[10] Williams B, MacDonald TM, Morant S, Webb DJ, Sever P, McInnes G, et al. Spironolactone versus placebo, bisoprolol, and doxazosin to determine the optimal treatment for drug-resistant hypertension (PATHWAY-2): a randomised, double-blind, crossover trial. Lancet. 2015;386:2059-68.

[11] Funder JW. Primary aldosteronism: clinical lateralization and costs. J Clin Endocrinol Metab. 2012;97:3450-2.

[12] Steichen O, Lorthioir A, Zinzindohoue F, Plouin P-F, Amar L. Outcomes of drug-based and surgical treatments for primary aldosteronism. Adv Chronic Kidney Dis. 2015;22:196-203.

[13] Ng L, Libertino JM. Adrenocortical carcinoma: diagnosis, evaluation and treatment. J Urol. 2003;169:5-11.

[14] Rossi GP. A comprehensive review of the clinical aspects of primary aldosteronism. Nat Rev Endocrinol. 2011;7:485-95.

[15] Solar M, Malirova E, Ballon M, Pelouch R, Ceral J. Confirmatory testing in primary aldosteronism: extensive medication switching is not needed in all patients. Eur J Endocrinol. 2012;166:679-86.

[16] Muth A, Ragnarsson O, Johannsson G, Wängberg B. Systematic review of surgery and outcomes in patients with primary aldosteronism. Br J Surg. 2015;102:307-17.

[17] Karagiannis A, Tziomalos K, Kakafika AI, Athyros VG, Harsoulis F, Mikhailidis DP. Medical treatment as an alternative to adrenalectomy in patients with aldosterone-producing adenomas. Endocr Relat Cancer. 2008;15:693-700.

[18] Marzano L, Colussi G, Sechi LA, Catena C. Adrenalectomy is comparable with medical treatment for reduction of left ventricular mass in primary aldosteronism: meta-analysis of long-term studies. Am J Hypertens. 2015;28:312-8.

[19] Catena C, Colussi G, Nadalini E, Chiuch A, Baroselli S, Lapenna R, et al. Cardiovascular outcomes in patients with primary aldosteronism after treatment. Arch Intern Med. 2008;168:80-5.

[20] Catena C, Lapenna R, Baroselli S, Nadalini E, Colussi G, Novello M, et al. Insulin sensitivity in patients with primary aldosteronism: a follow-up study. J Clin Endocrinol Metab. 2006;91:3457-63.

[21] Apostolopoulou K, Künzel HE, Gerum S, Merkle K, Schulz S, Fischer E, et al. Gender differences in anxiety and depressive symptoms in patients with primary hyperaldosteronism: a cross-sectional study. World J Biol Psychiatry. 2014;15:26-35.

[22] Fischer E, Beuschlein F, Degenhart C, Jung P, Bidlingmaier M, Reincke M. Spontaneous remission of idiopathic aldosteronism after long-term treatment with spironolactone: results from the German Conn's Registry. Clin Endocrinol (Oxf). 2012;76:473-7.

[23] Yoneda T, Demura M, Takata H, Kometani M, Karashima S, Yamagishi M, et al. Unilateral primary aldosteronism with spontaneous remission after long-term spironolactone therapy. J Clin Endocrinol Metab. 2012;97:1109-13.

[24] Kline GA, Pasieka JL, Harvey A, So B, Dias VC. Medical or surgical therapy for primary aldosteronism: post-treatment follow-up as a surrogate measure of comparative outcomes. Ann Surg Oncol. 2013;20:2274-8.

[25] Ahmed AH, Gordon RD, Sukor N, Pimenta E, Stowasser M. Quality of life in patients with bilateral primary aldosteronism before and during treatment with spironolactone and/or amiloride, including a comparison with our previously published results in those with unilateral disease treated surgically. J Clin Endocrinol Metab. 2011;96:2904-11.

[26] Stowasser M. Adrenal venous sampling for differentiating unilateral from bilateral primary aldosteronism: still the best, but could be better. Hypertension. 2015;65:704-6.

[27] Reimel B, Zanocco K, Russo MJ, Zarnegar R, Clark OH, Allendorf JD, et al. The management of aldosterone-producing adrenal adenomas – does adrenalectomy increase costs?. Surgery. 2010;148:1178-85; discussion 1185.

[28] Iacobone M, Citton M, Viel G, Rossi GP, Nitti D. Approach to the surgical management of primary aldosteronism. Gland Surg. 2015;4:69-81.

[29] Steichen O, Zinzindohoué F, Plouin P-F, Amar L. Outcomes of adrenalectomy in patients with unilateral primary aldosteronism: a review. Horm Metab Res. 2012;44:221-7.

[30] Iwakura Y, Ito S, Morimoto R, Kudo M, Ono Y, Nezu M, et al. Renal resistive index predicts postoperative blood pressure outcome in primary aldosteronism. Hypertension. 2016;67:654-60.

[31] Arnesen T, Glomnes N, Strømsøy S, Knappskog S, Heie A, Akslen LA, et al. Outcome after surgery for primary hyperaldosteronism may depend on KCNJ5 tumor mutation status: a population-based study from Western Norway. Langenbecks Arch Surg. 2013;398:869-74.

[32] Weigel M, Riester A, Hanslik G, Lang K, Willenberg HS, Endres S, et al. Post saline infusion test aldosterone levels indicate severity and outcome in primary aldosteronism. Eur J Endocrinol. 2015;172:443-50.

[33] Umakoshi H, Tanase-Nakao K, Wada N, Ichijo T, Sone M, Inagaki N, et al. Importance of contralateral aldosterone suppression during adrenal vein sampling in the subtype evaluation of primary aldosteronism. Clin Endocrinol (Oxf). 2015;83:462-7.

[34] Wolley MJ, Gordon RD, Ahmed AH, Stowasser M. Does contralateral suppression at adrenal venous sampling predict outcome following unilateral adrenalectomy for primary aldosteronism? A retrospective study. J Clin Endocrinol Metab. 2015;100:1477-84.

[35] Monticone S, Satoh F, Viola A, Fischer E, Vonend O, Bernini G, et al. Aldosterone suppression on contralateral adrenal during adrenal vein sampling does not predict blood pressure response after adrenalectomy. J Clin Endocrinol Metab. 2014;99:4158-66.

[36] Zarnegar R, Young WF, Lee J, Sweet MP, Kebebew E, Farley DR, et al. The aldosteronoma resolution score: predicting complete resolution of hypertension after adrenalectomy for aldosteronoma. Ann Surg. 2008;247:511-8.

[37] Utsumi T, Kamiya N, Endo T, Yano M, Kamijima S, Kawamura K, et al. Development of a novel nomogram to predict hypertension cure after laparoscopic adrenalectomy in patients with primary aldosteronism. World J Surg. 2014;38:2640-4.

[38] Kempers MJ, Lenders JW, van Outheusden L, van der Wilt GJ, Kool LJS, Hermus AR, et al. Systematic review: diagnostic procedures to differentiate unilateral from bilateral adrenal abnormality in primary aldosteronism. Ann Intern Med. 2009;151:329-37.

[39] Omura M, Sasano H, Fujiwara T, Yamaguchi K, Nishikawa T. Unique cases of unilateral hyperaldosteronemia due to multiple adrenocortical micronodules, which can only be detected by selective adrenal venous sampling. Metabolism. 2002;51:350-5.

[40] Dekkers T, Prejbisz A, Kool LJS, Groenewoud HJMM, Velema M, Spiering W, et al. Adrenal vein sampling versus CT scan to determine treatment in primary aldosteronism: an outcome-based randomised diagnostic trial. Lancet Diabetes Endocrinol. 2016;4:739-46.

[41] Reincke M. Adrenal vein sampling for subtyping in primary aldosteronism. Lancet Diabetes Endocrinol. 2016;4:718-9.

[42] Young WF. Minireview: primary aldosteronism--changing concepts in diagnosis and treatment. Endocrinology. 2003;144:2208-13.

[43] Betz MJ, Degenhart C, Fischer E, Pallauf A, Brand V, Linsenmaier U, et al. Adrenal vein sampling using rapid cortisol assays in primary aldosteronism is useful in centers with low success rates. Eur J Endocrinol. 2011;165:301-6.

[44] Park SI, Rhee Y, Lim JS, Park S, Kang SW, Lee MS, et al. Right adrenal venography findings correlated with C-arm CT for selection during C-arm CT-assisted adrenal vein sampling in primary aldosteronism. Cardiovasc Intervent Radiol. 2014;37:1469-75.

[45] Young WF, Stanson AW. What are the keys to successful adrenal venous sampling (AVS) in patients with primary aldosteronism?. Clin Endocrinol (Oxf). 2009;70:14-7.

[46] Daunt N. Adrenal vein sampling: how to make it quick, easy, and successful. Radiographics. 2005;25 Suppl 1:S143-58.

[47] Rossi GP, Barisa M, Allolio B, Auchus RJ, Amar L, Cohen D, et al. The Adrenal Vein Sampling International Study (AVIS) for identifying the major subtypes of primary aldosteronism. J Clin Endocrinol Metab. 2012;97:1606-14.

[48] Lethielleux G, Amar L, Raynaud A, Plouin P-F, Steichen O. Influence of diagnostic criteria on the interpretation of adrenal vein sampling. Hypertension. 2015;65:849-54.

[49] Monticone S, Viola A, Rossato D, Veglio F, Reincke M, Gomez-Sanchez C, et al. Adrenal vein sampling in primary aldosteronism: towards a standardised protocol. Lancet Diabetes Endocrinol. 2015;3:296-303.

[50] Rossi GP, Auchus RJ, Brown M, Lenders JWM, Naruse M, Plouin PF, et al. An expert consensus statement on use of adrenal vein sampling for the subtyping of primary aldosteronism. Hypertension. 2014;63:151-60.

[51] Rossi GP, Bernini G, Caliumi C, Desideri G, Fabris B, Ferri C, et al. A prospective study of the prevalence of primary aldosteronism in 1,125 hypertensive patients. J Am Coll Cardiol. 2006;48:2293-300.

[52] Mulatero P, Bertello C, Rossato D, Mengozzi G, Milan A, Garrone C, et al. Roles of clinical criteria, computed tomography scan, and adrenal vein sampling in differential diagnosis of primary aldosteronism subtypes. J Clin Endocrinol Metab. 2008;93:1366-71.

[53] Mulatero P, Milan A, Fallo F, Regolisti G, Pizzolo F, Fardella C, et al. Comparison of confirmatory tests for the diagnosis of primary aldosteronism. J Clin Endocrinol Metab. 2006;91:2618-23.

[54] Holland OB, Brown H, Kuhnert L, Fairchild C, Risk M, Gomez-Sanchez CE. Further evaluation of saline infusion for the diagnosis of primary aldosteronism. Hypertension. 1984;6:717-23.

[55] Rossi GP, Belfiore A, Bernini G, Desideri G, Fabris B, Ferri C, et al. Prospective evaluation of the saline infusion test for excluding primary aldosteronism due to aldosterone-producing adenoma. J Hypertens. 2007;25:1433-42.

[56] Nanba K, Tsuiki M, Umakoshi H, Nanba A, Hirokawa Y, Usui T, et al. Shortened saline infusion test for subtype prediction in primary aldosteronism. Endocrine. 2015;50:802-6.

[57] Sonoyama T, Sone M, Miyashita K, Tamura N, Yamahara K, Park K, et al. Significance of adrenocorticotropin stimulation test in the diagnosis of an aldosterone-producing adenoma. J Clin Endocrinol Metab. 2011;96:2771-8.

[58] Jiang Y, Zhang C, Wang W, Su T, Zhou W, Jiang L, et al. Diagnostic value of ACTH stimulation test in determining the subtypes of primary aldosteronism. J Clin Endocrinol Metab. 2015;100:1837-44.

[59] Satoh F, Morimoto R, Ono Y, Iwakura Y, Omata K, Kudo M, et al. Measurement of peripheral plasma 18-oxocortisol can discriminate unilateral adenoma from bilateral diseases in patients with primary aldosteronism. Hypertension. 2015;65:1096-102.

[60] Eisenhofer G, Dekkers T, Peitzsch M, Dietz AS, Bidlingmaier M, Treitl M, et al. Mass spectrometry-based adrenal and peripheral venous steroid profiling for subtyping primary aldosteronism. Clin Chem. 2016;62:514-24.

[61] Burton TJ, Mackenzie IS, Balan K, Koo B, Bird N, Soloviev DV, et al. Evaluation of the sensitivity and specificity of (11)C-metomidate positron emission tomography (PET)-CT for lateralizing aldosterone secretion by Conn's adenomas. J Clin Endocrinol Metab. 2012;97:100-9.

[62] Abe T, Naruse M, Young WF, Kobashi N, Doi Y, Izawa A, et al. A novel CYP11B2-specific imaging agent for detection of unilateral subtypes of primary aldosteronism. J Clin Endocrinol Metab. 2016;101:1008-15.

[63] Küpers EM, Amar L, Raynaud A, Plouin P-F, Steichen O. A clinical prediction score to diagnose unilateral primary aldosteronism. J Clin Endocrinol Metab. 2012;97:3530-7.

[64] Riester A, Fischer E, Degenhart C, Reiser MF, Bidlingmaier M, Beuschlein F, et al. Age below 40 or a recently proposed clinical prediction score cannot bypass adrenal venous sampling in primary aldosteronism. J Clin Endocrinol Metab. 2014;99:E1035-9.

[65] Venos ES, So B, Dias VC, Harvey A, Pasieka JL, Kline GA. A clinical prediction score for diagnosing unilateral primary Aldosteronism may not be generalizable. BMC Endocr Disord. 2014;14:94.

[66] Sze WCC, Soh LM, Lau JH, Reznek R, Sahdev A, Matson M, et al. Diagnosing unilateral primary aldosteronism - comparison of a clinical prediction score, computed tomography and adrenal venous sampling. Clin Endocrinol (Oxf). 2014;81:25-30.

[67] Nanba K, Tsuiki M, Nakao K, Nanba A, Usui T, Tagami T, et al. A subtype prediction score for primary aldosteronism. J Hum Hypertens. 2014;28:716-20.

[68] Kocjan T, Janez A, Stankovic M, Vidmar G, Jensterle M. A new clinical prediction criterion accurately determines a subset of patients with bilateral primary aldosteronism before adrenal venous sampling. Endocr Pract. 2016;22:587-94.

[69] Young WF, Stanson AW, Thompson GB, Grant CS, Farley DR, van Heerden JA. Role for adrenal venous sampling in primary aldosteronism. Surgery. 2004;136:1227-35.

[70] Lim V, Guo Q, Grant CS, Thompson GB, Richards ML, Farley DR, et al. Accuracy of adrenal imaging and adrenal venous sampling in predicting surgical cure of primary aldosteronism. J Clin Endocrinol Metab. 2014;99:2712-9.

Chapter 5

Pheochromocytomas

Helen M. Heneghan and Ruth S. Prichard

Additional information is available at the end of the chapter

http://dx.doi.org/10.5772/67373

Abstract

Pheochromocytomas are rare catecholamine-secreting neuroendocrine tumors derived from chromaffin tissue of the adrenal medulla. Such tumors arising from the sympathetic ganglia of the thorax, abdomen, or pelvis are termed "paragangliomas" or "extra-adrenal pheochromocytomas." The classic symptoms of these tumors are due to excess circulating levels of norepinephrine, epinephrine, or dopamine. Although 21% may be asymptomatic, the most common symptoms associated with pheochromocytomas include sweating, palpitations, and headaches in association with intermittent hypertension. If left untreated, excess catecholamines may result in hypertensive crisis leading to cardiac complications, cerebrovascular stroke, or ultimately sudden death. These catecholamine-secreting tumors are most commonly sporadic, but about 30% of patients have this disease as part of a familial disorder such as multiple endocrine neoplasia type 2 (MEN2) or von Hippel-Lindau (VHL) syndrome. Although most are benign, accurate recognition of pheochromocytomas with malignant potential and distant metastases remains a major diagnostic challenge. Advances in the field of molecular genetics have led to novel diagnostic and therapeutic strategies in an attempt to address this dilemma. Surgical excision of pheochromocytomas and paragangliomas is the mainstay of treatment and offers the only potential for cure. This chapter focuses on recent developments in the diagnosis of pheochromocytomas, encompassing biochemical, radiologic, histologic, and molecular analyzes. In addition, novel therapeutic strategies and advances in individualized targeted therapies for malignant pheochromocytomas will be discussed.

Keywords: pheochromocytoma, paraganglioma, diagnosis, management, therapeutics

1. Introduction

Pheochromocytomas are catecholamine-secreting tumors that arise from chromaffin cells of the adrenal medulla. Extra-adrenal pheochromocytomas or "paragangliomas" are those catecholamine-secreting tumors, which arise from the sympathetic ganglia. Whereas adrenal and extra-adrenal pheochromocytomas present and are treated similarly, the distinction between them is important for risk for malignancy, implications for associated neoplasms, and genetic testing. These rare neoplasms have an estimated annual incidence of approximately 0.8 per 100,000 person-years, and among people with hypertension in an outpatient setting, the prevalence varies between 0.2 and 0.6% [1–3]. Additionally, other tumors are discovered on autopsy such that the prevalence is likely to be underestimated [4]. The incidence of hereditary pheochromocytomas is estimated to be >30% in affected lineages [5]. Hereditary pheochromocytomas have been associated with >10 different germline mutations and are frequently a feature of a familial disorder or tumor syndrome, all of which have autosomal dominant inheritance (**Table 1**). They are also more likely to be malignant and bilateral than sporadic pheochromocytomas and present at younger ages.

Although pheochromocytomas may occur at any age, sporadic tumors are most common in the fourth to fifth decade, and there is no sex predilection [6]. The majority of pheochromocytomas and paragangliomas are benign and are associated with a normal life expectancy following treatment [7]. The incidence of malignancy is difficult to determine but ranges from 2.4 to 50% and higher among abdominal paragangliomas and those tumors harboring SDHB gene mutations [8–10]. Malignant pheochromocytomas often demonstrate local invasion, metastases, or recurrence and carry a worse prognosis with five-year survival rates of 20–70% [10–14].

Gene	Syndrome	Penetrance	Frequency of malignancy	PCC/PGL characteristics	Associated tumors
VHL	Von Hippel-Lindau	Autosomal dominant Variable expression	<10%	Young age (mean 28) Bilateral/multifocal	Retinal angiomas Hemangioblastoma Clear cell RCC
NF1	Neurofibromatosis	Autosomal dominant	<10%	Mean age 41 Bilateral disease common Extra adrenal PGL rare	Neurofibroma Neurofibrosarcoma Glioma Astrocytoma Carcinoid Leukemia
RET	MEN II	Autosomal dominant	<5% Extra-adrenal PGL rare	Mean age 40 Hyperparathyroidism No increased malignancy risk	Medullary thyroid cancer Mucosal neuromas
SDHC	PGL 3	Autosomal dominant	<5%	Mean age 46 Extra adrenal head & neck PGLs Bilateral/multifocal	Amyloidosis Cutaneous lichen GISTs

http://dx.doi.org/10.5772/67373

Gene	Syndrome	Penetrance	Frequency of malignancy	PCC/PGL characteristics	Associated tumors
SDHD	PGL 4	Autosomal dominant with parent of origin effect	<5%	Mean age 35 Extra adrenal head & neck PGLs Bilateral/multifocal	Papillary thyroid cancer GISTs
SDHB	PGL 1	Autosomal dominant	34–70%	Extra adrenal Increased malignancy risk Bilateral if adrenal	RCCs GISTs
SDHAF2	PGL 2	Autosomal dominant with parent of origin effect	Uncertain Head and neck PGLs	Extra adrenal	GISTs
TMEM 127		Autosomal dominant	5%	Adrenal Bilateral	
MAX		Autosomal dominant	10%	Adrenal Bilateral	

MEN, multiple endocrine neoplasia; PCC, pheochromocytoma; PGL, paraganglioma; RCC, renal cell carcinoma; GIST, gastrointestinal stromal tumor.

Table 1. Genetic mutations associated with pheochromocytomas and paragangliomas.

2. Clinical presentation

Since >50% of patients with pheochromocytomas are asymptomatic, these adrenal tumors are often identified as an "incidentaloma" on imaging studies obtained for other medical reasons or in patients with one of the hereditary syndromes of which pheochromocytomas are a feature. Symptoms reflect excessive secretion of norepinephrine, epinephrine, or dopamine into the circulation, and they are typically paroxysmal. The known triad of episodic headaches, sweating, and tachycardia occurs in about 40% of patients, although the majority will have two of these three classic symptoms [15]. Generalized sweating occurs in up to 70% of symptomatic patients. Other symptoms include palpitations, tremor, pallor, dyspnea, generalized weakness, and panic attack-type symptoms. Rarely, pheochromocytomas may present with a new diagnosis of diabetes, more commonly seen in younger patients who have no known risk factors. Approximately 50% of patients have paroxysmal hypertension, about 35–40% primary hypertension, and 10–15% are normotensive. A rare presentation due to an excess of circulating catecholamines, hypertensive crisis can precipitate life-threatening cardiovascular emergencies such as a myocardial infarction, cardiomyopathy, or a cerebrovascular accident in patients with pheochromoctyomas. Most common stimuli for eliciting hypertensive crises are exercise, tumor manipulation, and/or anesthesia, and for this reason, optimal preoperative and intraoperative management are essential [16].

Historically, pheochromocytomas and paragangliomas were thought to obey the "Rule of 10s": 10% malignant, 10% bilateral, 10% hereditary, 10% extra-adrenal, 10% children, 10% nonhypertensive, and 10% calcified. However, this rule does not appear to hold true anymore, with recent advances in molecular biology demonstrating that >50% of tumors have a genetic link, 50% of tumors have malignant potential, and 25% of tumors arise in an extra-adrenal location [17].

3. Hereditary pheochromocytomas: genetics

Pheochromocytomas have the strongest genetic component of endocrine tumors with up to 50% being linked to germline and somatic mutations in 17 different genes [18]. The rate of genetic association is higher in children who develop pheochromocytomas with rates of up to 69% (**Table 1**) [19]. Other genetic conditions such as the Carney triad and Carney-Stratakis syndrome are known to be associated with development of paragangliomas, but the underlying gene has not yet been identified. Multiple endocrine neoplasia type 2 (MEN 2) syndrome, subclassified into MEN 2A and MEN 2B, is associated with mutations in the tyrosine kinase receptor proto-oncogene RET. Patients affected with MEN 2 typically present with medullary thyroid cancer (MTC), and 50% will also have or develop pheochromocytomas. While half of these patients will have bilateral tumors, malignant transformation is rare [13, 20]. Patients with known MEN 2 now commonly undergo prophylactic total thyroidectomy and have ongoing imaging surveillance for development of a pheochromocytoma. As with MEN 2, von Hippel Lindau (VHL) and neurofibromatosis type 1 (NF1) are characterized by a predisposition to multiple tumor types. The rate of pheochromocytoma development in NF1 is significantly lower than in VHL or MEN 2 syndromes; however, the metastatic rate for NF1-associated pheochromocytomas of approximately 12% is higher than with MEN 2 or VHL [21]. The Carney Syndrome (or Carney Complex) is a triad of tumors, which includes the development of paragangliomas. First described in 1977, this complex includes the occurrence of pulmonary chondroma, gastrointestinal stromal tumors, and functioning paragangliomas in affected young women [22]. Carney-Stratakis syndrome is the association of familial paraganglioma with gastric stromal sarcomas. It is considered to be a distinct condition from the Carney Complex as it is not associated with pulmonary chondroma, and it exhibits an autosomal dominant pattern of inheritance [23].

Up to 25% of apparent sporadic cases result from germline loss-of-function mutations in the genes encoding the subunits A[F2], B, C, and D of succinate dehydrogenase (SDH) [24–27]. The SDH enzyme is involved in the Krebs cycle, where it catalyzes the oxidation of succinate to fumarate and also in the respiratory electron transfer chain, where it transfers electrons to coenzyme-Q. Germline mutations in the SDH gene complex give rise to the hereditary paraganglioma (PGL) and pheochromocytoma syndromes of which there are four. These syndromes are termed PGL1, PGL2, PGL3, and PGL4 and are attributable to mutations in SDHD, SDHAF2, SDHC, and SDHB, respectively [28]. In addition, germline mutations in the SDH gene have been identified in other hereditary paraganglioma syndromes such as Carney-Stratakis syndrome [29], whereas SDHB mutations are found in approximately 1.7–6.7% of sporadic pheochromocytomas and linked to more aggressive thoracic or intra-abdominal paragangliomas with younger age of presentation, multiple tumors, and higher metastatic rates [30]. SDH-related tumors are typically extra-adrenal, although some cases of adrenal pheochromocytomas have been reported. These patients also have an increased risk of renal cell carcinoma, which can have a more aggressive phenotype earlier in life [31].

http://dx.doi.org/10.5772/67373

Due to rapid developments in molecular research over the past decade, several additional genes have been identified that contribute to hereditary pheochromocytomas. These include myc-associated factor X (MAX) mutations that have been identified in this gene in 1.12% of patients with no other known mutations [32], transmembrane protein 127 (TMEM127) [33], and most recently, hypoxia-inducible factor 2-alpha (HIF2A) [34]. Genetic testing in patients with pheochromocytomas is an important component of management, although not routinely performed in most sporadic cases, as it is both expensive and time-consuming. A study using next-generation sequencing of pheochromocytomas that analyzes multiple genes simultaneously has proven highly sensitive in detecting mutations and may provide clinically relevant data in the future [35]. More patients with pheochromocytomas are being referred for next-generation sequencing with the goal of optimizing surveillance protocols and identifying family members at risk of developing pheochromocytoma for screening.

4. Diagnosis

4.1. Biochemical investigation

The diagnosis of pheochromocytoma is primarily made through biochemical investigations with subsequent anatomic and functional imaging delineating extent of disease. Guidelines from the Endocrine Society, European Society of Endocrinology, and American Association of Clinical Endocrinologists recommend the measurement of plasma or urinary fractionated metanephrines (specifically, the O-methylated metabolites of catecholamines), as they are most accurate for diagnosis of pheochromocytoma, demonstrating excellent sensitivity (97%) and specificity (91%) [2]. Metanephrines are consistently elevated in patients with biochemically active or functional pheochromocytomas despite fluctuating catecholamine release. When measuring 24-hour urinary metanephrines, urinary creatinine should also be measured to verify completeness of urine collection. For plasma metanephrine measurement, it is recommended that patients be in the supine position at least 30 min before blood is drawn [2]. It is also important prior to testing that any substances that may cause false-positive elevations in urinary or plasma metanephrine levels are discontinued, which includes certain antihypertensives, antidepressants (particularly levodopa, tricyclic antidepressants, and selective serotonin reuptake inhibitors (SSRI)), and caffeine. If these ideal testing conditions are not met, false-positive rates can be as high as 41% [36]. Diagnostic levels of metanephrines for pheochromocytoma are defined as levels greater than three times the upper reference limit. In patients with elevated metanephrines, but to a level less than the diagnostic threshold, urinary collection for metanephrines should be repeated to ensure correct conditions as stated above. If equivocal levels are confirmed, further biochemical tests are required that include a clonidine suppression test, in which plasma normetanephrine levels will remain elevated in the presence of a functioning pheochromocytoma or paraganglioma [37]. In patients considered to be low risk for pheochromoctyomas, measuring plasma fractionated metanephrines is the first-line investigation as the predictive value of a negative test is extremely high and excludes such tumors, except in patients with early preclinical disease. If metanephrine levels are normal in asymptomatic patients, then no further evaluation is necessary unless patients have typical paroxysmal symptoms in which biochemical testing should be repeated during a spell. In this scenario, patients are instructed to start a 24-hour urine collection when they have a typical spell. If results are still normal on repeat testing, other causes of spells should be investigated.

More recent studies have demonstrated the utility of plasma methoxytyramine in the diagnosis of pheochromocytoma, particularly for detecting exclusively dopamine-secreting tumors, which are rare and therefore can sometimes be overlooked by measuring only metanephrines [38, 39]. Chromogranin A, a polypeptide secreted by chromaffin cells, is the most accurate general biomarker for neuroendocrine tumors. Although not used in routine clinical practice, largely due to cost, chromogranin A is elevated in 91% of pheochromocytoma patients. While less specific, chromogranin A may be a valuable tool in monitoring response to treatment [40]. When chromogranin A is combined with catecholamine measurements, the sensitivity for diagnosis of pheochromocytoma approaches 100% and, in the majority of cases, normalizes after surgical resection of such tumors.

4.2. Radiologic studies

Once biochemical diagnosis of pheochromocytoma has been made, further evaluation with imaging is indicated to localize the primary tumor and assess for distant disease and allow for treatment planning including surgical resection. CT or MRI of the abdomen is initially performed to assess the adrenal gland. If these studies do not show an adrenal lesion in the presence of abnormal biochemical tests, then further imaging of the body is warranted [41]. CT and MRI are equally sensitive (98–100%) and specific (approximately 70%), and imaging choice depends upon cost, availability, and other issues such as radiation dose and use of contrast material. Historic concerns about contrast material provoking catecholamine release, and hypertensive crises have not been borne out in the literature; nonionic or low-osmolar contrast-enhanced CT is considered safe and does not require pretreatment with alpha- and beta-blockade [42]. The Endocrine Society recommends CT as the first-choice imaging modality because of its excellent spatial resolution for thorax, abdomen, and pelvis (**Figure 1**). MRI is the imaging modality of choice in patients with metastatic disease, head, and neck paragangliomas, CT-contrast allergies, pregnant women, children, and patients in whom radiation exposure should be limited (**Figure 2**) [2].

Functional imaging including metaiodobenzylguanidine scintigraphy (MIBG), positron emission tomography (PET), or somatostatin receptor imaging may also be required to evaluate the extent of disease, looking predominantly for extra-adrenal glands, and to accurately stage patients. Functional imaging is also indicated when abdominal CT or MRI is negative in the presence of clinical and biochemical evidence of pheochromocytoma. MIBG scintigraphy, using the catecholamine precursor 123I- or 131I-metaiodobenzylguanidine that is taken up by adrenergic tissue, is the first-line functional imaging modality. MIBG is a compound resembling norepinephrine that is taken up by adrenergic tissue. MIBG can identify tumors not detected by CT or MRI, in addition to localizing multiple or extra-adrenal tumors when CT or MRI abdomen is positive (**Figure 3**). Overall reported sensitivity and specificity of MIBG scanning is 94 and 92%, respectively [20]. Patients taking certain medications including tricyclic antidepressants, labetalol, and specific calcium antagonists should temporarily discontinue these drugs prior to scanning as they may interfere with 123I-MIBG uptake and image interpretation. 123I-MIBG has superior imaging quality than 131I-MIBG, and it is the radiotracer of choice when available

http://dx.doi.org/10.5772/67373

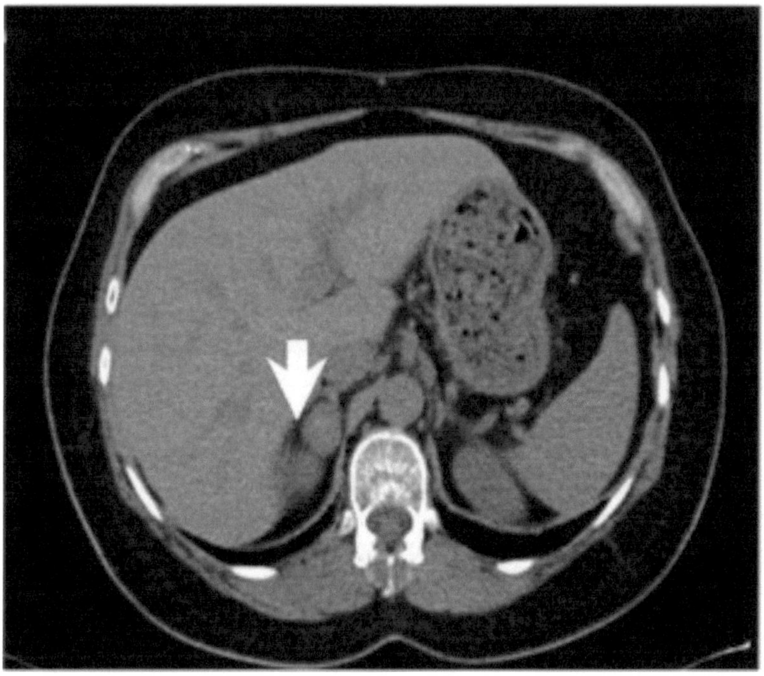

Figure 1. Axial CT imaging of a right adrenal heterogeneous mass measuring 34 hounsfield units on noncontrast phase. On enhanced and delayed series, the mass demonstrated relatively little washout and CT features are consistent for a pheochromocytoma.

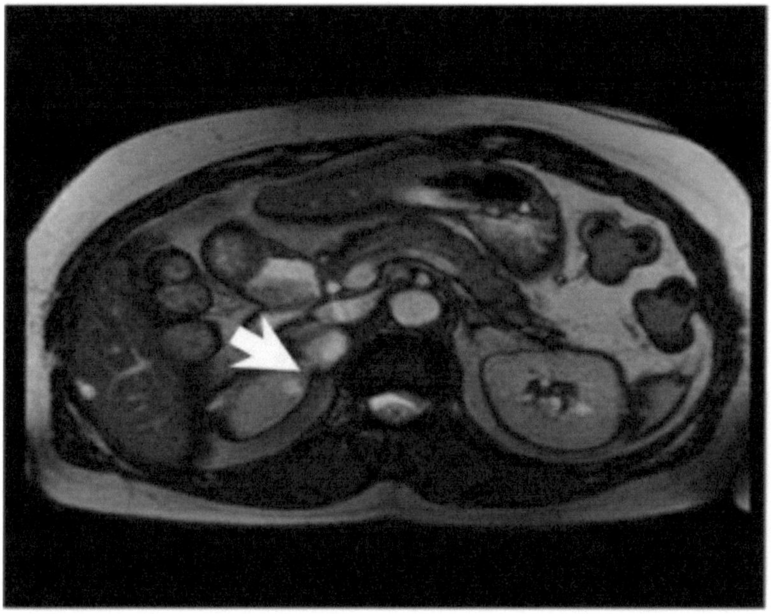

Figure 2. Axial MRI showing a mass (*white arrow*) in the medial limb of the right adrenal gland with a heterogeneously high signal on T2-weighted imaging consistent for a pheochromocytoma.

[43, 44]. A note of caution with regard to MIBG imaging is that its sensitivity is decreased in malignant pheochromocytomas [45]. This may be due to reduced expression of norepinephrine transporters in malignant adrenal tumors or dedifferentiation. It has been shown that tumors associated with VHL and SDHB genetic mutations may express a reduced number of noradrenaline transporters and, therefore, are more likely to be negative on MIBG imaging [46, 47].

Single-photon emission computed tomography (SPECT) imaging has been used in combination with both CT and MRI to increase accuracy in tumor localization as it involves simultaneous acquisition of both morphologic and functional data (**Figure 4**). However, SPECT imaging can miss smaller lesions due to relatively low resolution. Positron emission tomography (PET), using biologically active tracer-labeled molecules (18F-flurodeoxyglucose (FDG) most commonly), is increasingly employed in the diagnostic workup of pheochromocytomas and paragangliomas, particularly in patients where MIBG is negative. Although the 18F-FDG tracer is not specific for pheochromocytomas, it is useful in detecting pheochromocytomas and paragangliomas that do not accumulate MIBG, and it is superior to other functional imaging techniques in patients with disease associated with SDHB mutations [46]. The Endocrine Society guidelines favor [18F-FDG] PET-CT as the preferred imaging modality over 123I-MIBG scintigraphy in patients with known metastatic disease [2]. Recently, more specific tracers including 18F-DOPA, 18F-FDA (fluorodopamine), and 11C-HED (metahydroxephedrine) have been developed for pheochromocytoma and paraganglioma functional imaging but are not yet widely available.

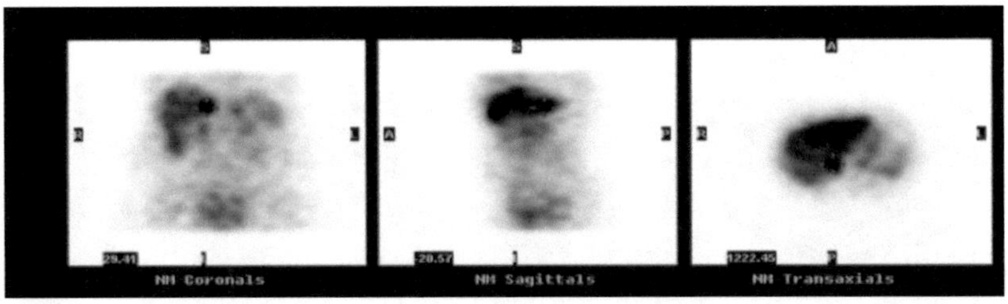

Figure 3. ^{123}I-MIBG scan showing focal uptake in the right adrenal gland consistent for a pheochromocytoma.

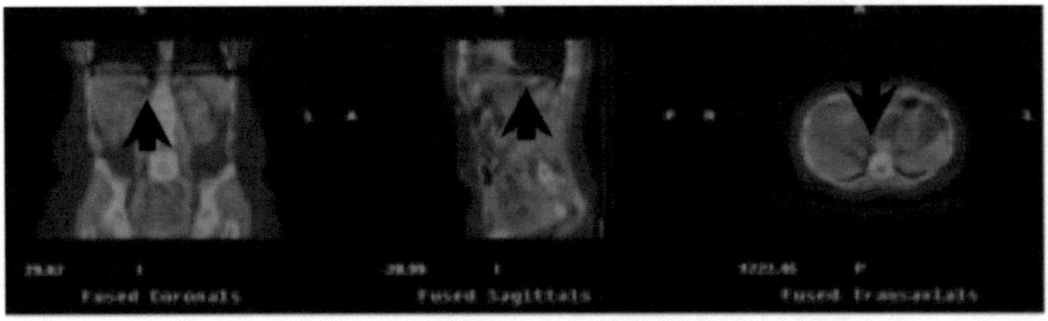

Figure 4. SPECT/CT imaging demonstrates focal tracer uptake in the right suprarenal region (*arrow*) suspicious for a right adrenal pheochromocytoma.

Image-guided needle biopsy of suspected pheochromocytomas should be avoided due to a high rate of biopsy-related complications such as triggering hypertensive crises, hematoma, severe pain, incorrect or inadequate biopsy, increased difficulty of surgical resection, and delay to definitive surgical treatment [48].

4.3. Histopathologic diagnosis of pheochromocytoma

The histologic diagnosis of pheochromocytomas is rather uncomplicated but difficulty arises when differentiating benign from malignant tumors. Tumor cells in pheochromocytomas and paragangliomas demonstrate a typical nested Zellballen pattern surrounded by sustentacular cells, which stain positive for S100 protein on immunohistochemistry. Characteristically, they exhibit immunopositivity for synaptophysin and chromogranin A and may express neurofilament [49]. There are no absolute histologic criteria for the diagnosis of malignancy and no reliable means to identify patients with pheochromocytomas who are at the risk of recurrence or metastatic spread using standard histopathologic techniques. Several histologic scoring systems have been devised to guide pathologists in the diagnosis of malignancy. The pheochromocytoma of the adrenal gland scoring system (PASS), devised by Thompson in 2002, is the most commonly used system (**Table 2**) [50]. In PASS, the histologic features of each pheochromocytoma are given a score, and the sum score is used to stratify the tumors into groups with potential for aggressive behavior (PASS > 4) and those likely to behave in a benign manner (PASS < 4). It is recommended that any patient with a PASS score of >4 should be closely followed [51]. However, this scoring system has limitations. It has been shown to have significant interobserver and intraobserver variation leading to recommendations that it be used with caution.

Features	Score
Large nest of cells or diffuse growth >10% of tumor volume	2
Necrosis (confluent or central in large nests)	2
High cellularity	2
Cellular monotony	2
Presence of spindle shaped tumor cells	2
Atypical mitotic figures (>3 per 10 high power fields)	2
Extension of tumor into adjacent fat	2
Vascular invasion	1
Capsular invasion	1
Profound nuclear pleomorphism	1
Nuclear hyperchromasia	1

A PASS score of <4 suggest a pheochromocytoma likely to behave in a benign manner [50].
A PASS score of ≥4 indicates a tumor with potentially aggressive behavior (PASS ≥ 4).

Table 2. Pheochromocytoma of the adrenal gland scoring scale (PASS).

Although several immunohistochemical markers of malignancy for pheochromocytomas have been proposed, none have emerged as reliable candidates for routine use in clinical practice. Markers that have been investigated to date include neuroendocrine-related and catecholamine-related markers (neuropeptide Y, 3,4-dihydroxyphenylalanine), granin-derived peptides (EM66, secretogranin II), CD-44s, angiogenic markers, and regulators (vascular endothelial growth factor (VEGF) and VEGFR), heat shock protein 90, and telomerase complex proteins.

5. Treatment

The curative treatment of choice for pheochromocytomas is surgical resection. However, management of some pheochromocytomas (particularly malignant, metastatic, or recurrent tumors) requires a multimodal therapeutic approach including pharmacologic control of catecholamine-mediated symptoms, radiotherapy, and systemic chemotherapy [52].

5.1. Pharmacologic management

Antihypertensive medications should be initiated in patients with biochemically active pheochromocytomas, not only to manage symptoms, but also to reduce the risk of a hypertensive crisis that can have devastating consequences. Initial pharmacologic management involves alpha-adrenoceptor blockers (e.g., long-acting phenoxybenzamine or short-acting prazosin, terazosin, or doxazosin) followed by cardioselective beta-blockade (e.g., metoprolol or atenolol) when necessary for reflexive tachycardia. It is important not to initiate beta-blockers before alpha blockade as this can lead to unopposed stimulation of alpha-adrenoceptors resulting in a hypertensive crisis [53]. Other hypertensive medications including calcium channel blockers are occasionally prescribed for patients with refractory hypertension, as single agents in patients with mild hypertension or in those who cannot tolerate alpha blockade [54].

5.2. Pre-operative care

All patients with a known pheochromocytoma who are scheduled to undergo surgical resection should have an extensive preoperative evaluation to exclude underlying metastatic disease that, if present, may influence treatment approach. Preoperative pharmacologic blockade using appropriate antihypertensive medication and careful fluid resuscitation is imperative to reduce the possibility of intraoperative hypertensive crises [55]. It is recommended that even patients who are normotensive preoperatively should receive alpha and possible beta-blockade, as unanticipated catecholamine release by the tumor during surgery may still precipitate hypertensive crisis [53]. As the alpha-blocker dose is increased, patients should start to have symptoms such as stuffy nose, fatigue, and mild postural hypotension that reflect adequate blockade. All patients should have a comprehensive anesthetic clearance preoperatively to assess cardiorespiratory fitness for surgery. Endocrine

http://dx.doi.org/10.5772/67373

Society guidelines recommend a high sodium diet along with sufficient fluid intake to reverse catecholamine-induced blood volume contraction preoperatively to prevent severe hypotension following tumor removal [2]. Cardiovascular parameters and blood glucose should also be carefully monitored perioperatively.

5.3. Adrenalectomy

Adrenalectomy is the treatment of choice for pheochromocytomas [56]. A laparoscopic surgical approach is the current preferred technique when technically feasible (**Figure 5**). It is associated with shorter length of stay, decreased analgesic requirements, and increased patient satisfaction [9, 57]. There is no consensus yet with respect to the superior laparoscopic approach—transperitoneal or retroperitoneal; the choice is determined by the surgeon's experience and preference. In patients with bilateral pheochromoctyomas or those at risk of bilateral disease due to known syndromes such as MEN2 or VHL, bilateral cortical sparing adrenalectomy has been proposed [58]. It is important to consider underlying genotype when selecting patients suitable for cortical sparing adrenalectomy as patients with MEN-2A or VHL mutations have a high risk of bilateral tumors yet low rates of malignancy, whereas patients with SDHB mutations should undergo total adrenalectomy carried out due to the increased risk of malignancy associated with these mutations. Patients with extensive locoregional infiltration from malignant pheochromocytomas usually require an open procedure to remove the tumor and any involved organs *en bloc*. For patients in whom safe curative surgical excision is deemed impossible, debulking/cytoreductive surgery can improve symptoms caused by local invasion. For patients with benign pheochromocytomas, surgical excision alone is curative. However, for patients with suspected or confirmed metastatic disease, alternative or additional treatment modalities may be required.

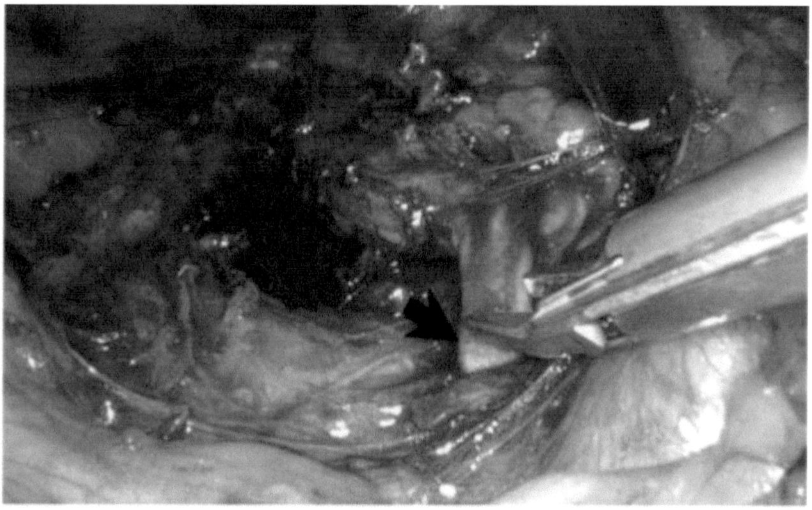

Figure 5. Transperitoneal laparoscopic left adrenalectomy showing the left adrenal vein (*arrow*) dissected prior to ligation.

5.4. Radiotherapy

Although malignant pheochromocytomas have limited radiosensitivity, patients with metastatic disease and those unsuitable for surgical intervention may be candidates for radiotherapy. Radiofrequency ablation and external beam radiotherapy are modalities in current use [59]. Radiotherapy is also used in the treatment of unresectable head and neck paragangliomas where long-term control can be obtained with limited toxicity [60]. When used in conjunction with radionuclide therapy (131I-MIBG), external radiation has been shown to improve response rates in a small number of patients with widespread systemic metastases [61].

5.5. Radionuclide therapy

Radionuclide treatment is indicated for patients with malignant disease in whom surgery is not a feasible option. Based on administration of radioactive compounds leading to the emission of beta particles into tumor cells causing their destruction, these beta-emitting isotopes are coupled to either 131I-MIBG or somatostatin analogs that allow uptake into chromaffin cells of adrenergic tissue. Patients with metastatic disease with 131I-MIBG uptake on imaging may be suitable for this treatment modality.

5.6. Chemotherapy

Malignant pheochromocytomas are not particularly chemosensitive. Chemotherapy is largely reserved for those patients not amenable to surgical therapy and who do not respond to radionuclide treatment. The most common regimen of cyclophosphamide, vincristine, and dacarbazine (CVD) has been shown to be of some value in palliating symptoms of advanced disease, reducing the rate of tumor growth, and occasionally decreasing tumor size [62, 63]. Experience with alternative chemotherapeutic agents for pheochromocytomas is limited and mostly based on isolated case reports and small series. Further, clinical trials are needed before recommendations can be made on their use in pheochromocytomas and paragangliomas [64].

5.7. Targeted therapy

Since standard adjuvant therapies have been demonstrated to have limited efficacy in treating advanced pheochromocytomas, newer therapeutic targets are currently being studied. Underlying genetic mutations and molecular alterations associated with malignancy have led to the identification of molecular therapeutic targets that include the mammalian rapamycin (mTOR) protein kinase, which is known to be upregulated in malignant pheochromocytomas [65], angiogenesis-mediated growth factors such as vascular endothelial growth factor (VEGF) and heat shock protein 90 (Hsp90), which are also overexpressed in malignant pheochromocytomas [66]. The mTOR inhibitor, Everolimus, has been used in a number of patients with malignant pheochromocytomas, but results have been disappointing [67]. This may be due to compensatory P13K/AKT and ERK activation in response to mTOR inhibition [68]. Further studies of targeting more than one pathway to overcome drug resistance are in progress using a combination of mTOR inhibition with other specific molecular drugs.

http://dx.doi.org/10.5772/67373

Like other tumors, targeting angiogenesis-mediated tumor growth by the VEGF pathway has been evaluated in the treatment of malignant pheochromocytoma. Sunitinib, a tyrosine kinase inhibitor that inhibits VEGF-R, PDGF, and c-KIT, was originally developed as a treatment for renal cell carcinoma but has shown some promising results for malignant pheochromocytomas with reduction in tumor size, catecholamine secretion, and metabolic activity on functional imaging [69]. Additional targets for therapy of pheochromocytomas will be identified with increasing understanding of tumor pathogenesis.

6. Summary

With the advent of improved diagnostic imaging and a greater understanding of molecular genetics, an increasing number of patients with pheochromocytomas are being identified. The majority of these patients have benign disease that can be cured by minimally invasive surgical resection. The recognition of malignant potential remains a major diagnostic challenge, and the presence of metastatic disease still carries a poor prognosis. Several targets for therapy have been already identified for further evaluation, which may offer promising therapeutic options in the future.

Author details

Helen M. Heneghan and Ruth S. Prichard*

*Address all correspondence to: ruthprichard@rcsi.ie

Department of Endocrine Surgery, St. Vincent's University Hospital, Dublin, Ireland

References

[1] Beard CM, Sheps SG, Kurland LT, Carney JA, Lie JT. Occurrence of pheochromocytoma in Rochester, Minnesota, 1950 through 1979. Mayo Clin Proc. 1983;58(12):802–4.

[2] Lenders JW, Duh QY, Eisenhofer G, Gimenez-Roqueplo AP, Grebe SK, Murad MH, et al. Pheochromocytoma and paraganglioma: an endocrine society clinical practice guideline. J Clin Endocrinol Metab. 2014;99(6):1915–42.

[3] Omura M, Saito J, Yamaguchi K, Kakuta Y, Nishikawa T. Prospective study on the prevalence of secondary hypertension among hypertensive patients visiting a general outpatient clinic in Japan. Hypertens Res Off J Jpn Soc Hypertens. 2004;27(3):193–202.

[4] Sutton MG, Sheps SG, Lie JT. Prevalence of clinically unsuspected pheochromocytoma. Review of a 50-year autopsy series. Mayo Clin Proc. 1981;56(6):354–60.

[5] Gimenez-Roqueplo AP, Dahia PL, Robledo M. An update on the genetics of paraganglioma, pheochromocytoma, and associated hereditary syndromes. Hormone and

Metabolic Research = Hormon- und Stoffwechselforschung = Hormones et metabolisme. 2012;44(5):328–33.

[6] Guerrero MA, Schreinemakers JM, Vriens MR, Suh I, Hwang J, Shen WT, et al. Clinical spectrum of pheochromocytoma. J Am Coll Surg. 2009;209(6):727–32.

[7] Timmers HJ, Brouwers FM, Hermus AR, Sweep FC, Verhofstad AA, Verbeek AL, et al. Metastases but not cardiovascular mortality reduces life expectancy following surgical resection of apparently benign pheochromocytoma. Endocr Relat Cancer. 2008; 15(4):1127–33.

[8] Proye C, Vix M, Goropoulos A, Kerlo P, Lecomte-Houcke M. High incidence of malignant pheochromocytoma in a surgical unit. 26 cases out of 100 patients operated from 1971 to 1991. J Endocrinol Invest. 1992;15(9):651–63.

[9] Walz MK, Alesina PF, Wenger FA, Koch JA, Neumann HP, Petersenn S, et al. Laparoscopic and retroperitoneoscopic treatment of pheochromocytomas and retroperitoneal paragangliomas: results of 161 tumors in 126 patients. World J Surg. 2006;30(5):899–908.

[10] Chrisoulidou A, Kaltsas G, Ilias I, Grossman AB. The diagnosis and management of malignant phaeochromocytoma and paraganglioma. Endocr Relat Cancer. 2007;14(3):569–85.

[11] Nomura K, Kimura H, Shimizu S, Kodama H, Okamoto T, Obara T, et al. Survival of patients with metastatic malignant pheochromocytoma and efficacy of combined cyclophosphamide, vincristine, and dacarbazine chemotherapy. J Clin Endocrinol Metab. 2009;94(8): 2850–6.

[12] Sisson JC, Shulkin BL, Esfandiari NH. Courses of malignant pheochromocytoma: implications for therapy. Ann N Y Acad Sci. 2006;1073:505–11.

[13] Tischler AS. Pheochromocytoma: time to stamp out "malignancy"?. Endocr Pathol. 2008;19(4):207–8.

[14] Zarnegar R, Kebebew E, Duh QY, Clark OH. Malignant pheochromocytoma. Surg Oncol Clin N Am. 2006;15(3):555–71.

[15] Soltani A, Pourian M, Davani BM. Does this patient have pheochromocytoma? a systematic review of clinical signs and symptoms. J Diabetes Metab Disord. 2015;15:6.

[16] Brouwers FM, Lenders JW, Eisenhofer G, Pacak K. Pheochromocytoma as an endocrine emergency. Rev Endocr Metab Disord. 2003;4(2):121–8.

[17] Madani R, Al-Hashmi M, Bliss R, Lennard TW. Ectopic pheochromocytoma: does the rule of tens apply?. World J Surg. 2007;31(4):849–54.

[18] Martucci VL, Pacak K. Pheochromocytoma and paraganglioma: diagnosis, genetics, management, and treatment. Curr Probl Cancer. 2014;38(1):7–41.

[19] Cascon A, Inglada-Perez L, Comino-Mendez I, de Cubas AA, Leton R, Mora J, et al. Genetics of pheochromocytoma and paraganglioma in Spanish pediatric patients. Endocr Relat Cancer. 2013;20(3):L1–6.

[20] Bombardieri E, Giammarile F, Aktolun C, Baum RP, Bischof Delaloye A, Maffioli L, et al. 131I/123I-metaiodobenzylguanidine (mIBG) scintigraphy: procedure guidelines for tumour imaging. Eur J Nucl Med Mol Imaging. 2010;37(12):2436–46.

[21] Karasek D, Shah U, Frysak Z, Stratakis C, Pacak K. An update on the genetics of pheochromocytoma. J Hum Hypertens. 2013;27(3):141–7.

[22] Carney JA, Sheps SG, Go VL, Gordon H. The triad of gastric leiomyosarcoma, functioning extra-adrenal paraganglioma and pulmonary chondroma. N Engl J Med. 1977;296(26):1517–8.

[23] Carney JA, Stratakis CA. Familial paraganglioma and gastric stromal sarcoma: a new syndrome distinct from the Carney triad. Am J Med Genet. 2002;108(2):132–9.

[24] Astuti D, Douglas F, Lennard TW, Aligianis IA, Woodward ER, Evans DG, et al. Germline SDHD mutation in familial phaeochromocytoma. Lancet. 2001;357(9263):1181–2.

[25] Baysal BE, Ferrell RE, Willett-Brozick JE, Lawrence EC, Myssiorek D, Bosch A, et al. Mutations in SDHD, a mitochondrial complex II gene, in hereditary paraganglioma. Science. 2000;287(5454):848–51.

[26] Neumann HP, Bausch B, McWhinney SR, Bender BU, Gimm O, Franke G, et al. Germ-line mutations in nonsyndromic pheochromocytoma. N Engl J Med. 2002;346(19):1459–66.

[27] Peczkowska M, Cascon A, Prejbisz A, Kubaszek A, Cwikla BJ, Furmanek M, et al. Extra-adrenal and adrenal pheochromocytomas associated with a germline SDHC mutation. Nat Clin Pract Endocrinol Metab. 2008;4(2):111–5.

[28] Ricketts C, Woodward ER, Killick P, Morris MR, Astuti D, Latif F, et al. Germline SDHB mutations and familial renal cell carcinoma. J Natl Cancer Inst. 2008;100(17):1260–2.

[29] Pasini B, McWhinney SR, Bei T, Matyakhina L, Stergiopoulos S, Muchow M, et al. Clinical and molecular genetics of patients with the Carney-Stratakis syndrome and germline mutations of the genes coding for the succinate dehydrogenase subunits SDHB, SDHC, and SDHD. Eur J Hum Genet. 2008;16(1):79–88.

[30] van Hulsteijn LT, Dekkers OM, Hes FJ, Smit JW, Corssmit EP. Risk of malignant paraganglioma in SDHB-mutation and SDHD-mutation carriers: a systematic review and meta-analysis. J Med Genet. 2012;49(12):768–76.

[31] Gill AJ, Pachter NS, Clarkson A, Tucker KM, Winship IM, Benn DE, et al. Renal tumors and hereditary pheochromocytoma-paraganglioma syndrome type 4. N Engl J Med. 2011;364(9):885–6.

[32] Burnichon N, Cascon A, Schiavi F, Morales NP, Comino-Mendez I, Abermil N, et al. MAX mutations cause hereditary and sporadic pheochromocytoma and paraganglioma. Clin Cancer Res. 2012;18(10):2828–37.

[33] Qin Y, Yao L, King EE, Buddavarapu K, Lenci RE, Chocron ES, et al. Germline mutations in TMEM127 confer susceptibility to pheochromocytoma. Nat Genet. 2010;42(3):229–33.

[34] Zhuang Z, Yang C, Lorenzo F, Merino M, Fojo T, Kebebew E, et al. Somatic HIF2A gain-of-function mutations in paraganglioma with polycythemia. N Engl J Med. 2012;367(10):922–30.

[35] Rattenberry E, Vialard L, Yeung A, Bair H, McKay K, Jafri M, et al. A comprehensive next generation sequencing-based genetic testing strategy to improve diagnosis of inherited pheochromocytoma and paraganglioma. J Clin Endocrinol Metab. 2013;98(7):E1248–56.

[36] Eisenhofer G, Goldstein DS, Walther MM, Friberg P, Lenders JW, Keiser HR, et al. Biochemical diagnosis of pheochromocytoma: how to distinguish true- from false-positive test results. J Clin Endocrinol Metab. 2003;88(6):2656–66.

[37] Eisenhofer G, Siegert G, Kotzerke J, Bornstein SR, Pacak K. Current progress and future challenges in the biochemical diagnosis and treatment of pheochromocytomas and paragangliomas. Horm Metab Res. 2008;40(5):329–37.

[38] Eisenhofer G, Goldstein DS, Sullivan P, Csako G, Brouwers FM, Lai EW, et al. Biochemical and clinical manifestations of dopamine-producing paragangliomas: utility of plasma methoxytyramine. J Clin Endocrinol Metab. 2005;90(4):2068–75.

[39] Poirier E, Thauvette D, Hogue JC. Management of exclusively dopamine-secreting abdominal pheochromocytomas. J Am Coll Surg. 2013;216(2):340–6.

[40] Grossrubatscher E, Dalino P, Vignati F, Gambacorta M, Pugliese R, Boniardi M, et al. The role of chromogranin A in the management of patients with phaeochromocytoma. Clin Endocrinol (Oxf). 2006;65(3):287–93.

[41] Taieb D, Timmers HJ, Hindie E, Guillet BA, Neumann HP, Walz MK, et al. EANM 2012 guidelines for radionuclide imaging of phaeochromocytoma and paraganglioma. Eur J Nucl Med Mol Imaging. 2012;39(12):1977–95.

[42] Baid SK, Lai EW, Wesley RA, Ling A, Timmers HJ, Adams KT, et al. Brief communication: radiographic contrast infusion and catecholamine release in patients with pheochromocytoma. Ann Intern Med. 2009;150(1):27–32.

[43] Furuta N, Kiyota H, Yoshigoe F, Hasegawa N, Ohishi Y. Diagnosis of pheochromocytoma using [123I]-compared with [131I]-metaiodobenzylguanidine scintigraphy. Int J Urol. 1999;6(3):119–24.

[44] Solanki KK, Bomanji J, Moyes J, Mather SJ, Trainer PJ, Britton KE. A pharmacological guide to medicines which interfere with the biodistribution of radiolabelled meta-iodobenzylguanidine (MIBG). Nucl Med Commun. 1992;13(7):513–21.

[45] Van Der Horst-Schrivers AN, Jager PL, Boezen HM, Schouten JP, Kema IP, Links TP. Iodine-123 metaiodobenzylguanidine scintigraphy in localising phaeochromocytomas—experience and meta-analysis. Anticancer Res. 2006;26(2B):1599–604.

[46] Fonte JS, Robles JF, Chen CC, Reynolds J, Whatley M, Ling A, et al. False-negative (1)(2)(3)I-MIBG SPECT is most commonly found in SDHB-related pheochromocytoma or paraganglioma with high frequency to develop metastatic disease. Endocr Relat Cancer. 2012;19(1):83–93.

[47] Kaji P, Carrasquillo JA, Linehan WM, Chen CC, Eisenhofer G, Pinto PA, et al. The role of 6-[18F]fluorodopamine positron emission tomography in the localization of adrenal pheochromocytoma associated with von Hippel-Lindau syndrome. Eur J Endocrinol. 2007;156(4):483–7.

[48] Vanderveen KA, Thompson SM, Callstrom MR, Young WF, Jr., Grant CS, Farley DR, et al. Biopsy of pheochromocytomas and paragangliomas: potential for disaster. Surgery. 2009;146(6):1158–66.

[49] Kimura N, Nakazato Y, Nagura H, Sasano N. Expression of intermediate filaments in neuroendocrine tumors. Arch Pathol Lab Med. 1990;114(5):506–10.

[50] Thompson LD. Pheochromocytoma of the adrenal gland scaled score (PASS) to separate benign from malignant neoplasms: a clinicopathologic and immunophenotypic study of 100 cases. Am J Surg Pathol. 2002;26(5):551–66.

[51] Strong VE, Kennedy T, Al-Ahmadie H, Tang L, Coleman J, Fong Y, et al. Prognostic indicators of malignancy in adrenal pheochromocytomas: clinical, histopathologic, and cell cycle/apoptosis gene expression analysis. Surgery. 2008;143(6):759–68.

[52] Pacak K, Eisenhofer G, Ahlman H, Bornstein SR, Gimenez-Roqueplo AP, Grossman AB, et al. Pheochromocytoma: recommendations for clinical practice from the first international symposium. October 2005. Nat Clin Pract Endocrinol Metab. 2007;3(2):92–102.

[53] Pacak K. Preoperative management of the pheochromocytoma patient. J Clin Endocrinol Metab. 2007;92(11):4069–79.

[54] Mazza A, Armigliato M, Marzola MC, Schiavon L, Montemurro D, Vescovo G, et al. Anti-hypertensive treatment in pheochromocytoma and paraganglioma: current management and therapeutic features. Endocrine. 2014;45(3):469–78.

[55] Adler JT, Meyer-Rochow GY, Chen H, Benn DE, Robinson BG, Sippel RS, et al. Pheochromocytoma: current approaches and future directions. Oncologist. 2008;13(7): 779–93.

[56] Lenders JW, Eisenhofer G, Mannelli M, Pacak K. Phaeochromocytoma. Lancet. 2005; 366(9486):665–75.

[57] Gumbs AA, Gagner M. Laparoscopic adrenalectomy. Best Pract Res Clin Endocrinol Metab. 2006;20(3):483–99.

[58] Brauckhoff M, Thanh PN, Gimm O, Bar A, Brauckhoff K, Dralle H. Functional results after endoscopic subtotal cortical-sparing adrenalectomy. Surg Today. 2003;33(5):342–8.

[59] Pappachan JM, Raskauskiene D, Sriraman R, Edavalath M, Hanna FW. Diagnosis and management of pheochromocytoma: a practical guide to clinicians. Curr Hypertens Rep. 2014;16(7):442.

[60] Chino JP, Sampson JH, Tucci DL, Brizel DM, Kirkpatrick JP. Paraganglioma of the head and neck: long-term local control with radiotherapy. Am J Clin Oncol. 2009;32(3):304–7.

[61] Fishbein L, Bonner L, Torigian DA, Nathanson KL, Cohen DL, Pryma D, et al. External beam radiation therapy (EBRT) for patients with malignant pheochromocytoma and non-head and -neck paraganglioma: combination with 131I-MIBG. Horm Metab Res. 2012;44(5):405–10.

[62] Jimenez C, Rohren E, Habra MA, Rich T, Jimenez P, Ayala-Ramirez M, et al. Current and future treatments for malignant pheochromocytoma and sympathetic paraganglioma. Curr Oncol Rep. 2013;15(4):356–71.

[63] Ayala-Ramirez M, Feng L, Habra MA, Rich T, Dickson PV, Perrier N, et al. Clinical benefits of systemic chemotherapy for patients with metastatic pheochromocytomas or sympathetic extra-adrenal paragangliomas: insights from the largest single-institutional experience. Cancer. 2012;118(11):2804–12.

[64] Fishbein L. Pheochromocytoma and paraganglioma: genetics, diagnosis, and treatment. Hematol Oncol Clin North Am. 2016;30(1):135–50.

[65] Yuan R, Kay A, Berg WJ, Lebwohl D. Targeting tumorigenesis: development and use of mTOR inhibitors in cancer therapy. J Hematol Oncol. 2009;2:45.

[66] Boltze C, Mundschenk J, Unger N, Schneider-Stock R, Peters B, Mawrin C, et al. Expression profile of the telomeric complex discriminates between benign and malignant pheochromocytoma. J Clin Endocrinol Metab. 2003;88(9):4280–6.

[67] Druce MR, Kaltsas GA, Fraenkel M, Gross DJ, Grossman AB. Novel and evolving therapies in the treatment of malignant phaeochromocytoma: experience with the mTOR inhibitor everolimus (RAD001). Horm Metab Res. 2009;41(9):697–702.

[68] Zitzmann K, Ruden J, Brand S, Goke B, Lichtl J, Spottl G, et al. Compensatory activation of Akt in response to mTOR and Raf inhibitors—a rationale for dual-targeted therapy approaches in neuroendocrine tumor disease. Cancer Lett. 2010;295(1):100–9.

[69] Ayala-Ramirez M, Chougnet CN, Habra MA, Palmer JL, Leboulleux S, Cabanillas ME, et al. Treatment with sunitinib for patients with progressive metastatic pheochromocytomas and sympathetic paragangliomas. J Clin Endocrinol Metab. 2012;97(11):4040–50.

Chapter 6

Pheochromocytoma Crisis

Tanya Castelino and Elliot Mitmaker

Additional information is available at the end of the chapter

http://dx.doi.org/10.5772/intechopen.69338

Abstract

Pheochromocytomas are rare tumours of the adrenal gland that secrete catecholamines. The classical presentation of these tumours consists of a clinical triad of headaches, palpitations and diaphoresis. This clinical presentation should not be confused with the potentially fatal presentation of pheochromocytoma crisis, which may include severe haemodynamic instability and collapse, multi-organ failure, hyperthermia and encephalopathy. When patients present in profound shock, supportive care and treatment are initiated. Patients presenting with pheochromocytoma crisis have an underlying adrenal tumour, but the clinical manifestations of this life-threatening condition can mimic other entities. Once diagnosis is made, previous anecdotal evidence has shown that pheochromocytoma crisis is a surgical emergency. However, retrospective study of a larger sample of patients presenting with pheochromocytoma crisis suggests that medical management in the acute setting is appropriate and safe. The ultimate treatment is indeed surgical; however, there is no clear recommendation for the acute management of pheochromocytoma crisis. This chapter will focus on the medical and surgical management of potentially life-threatening pheochromocytoma crisis. An in-depth review of the clinical presentation, pathophysiology, causes and treatments of pheochromocytoma crisis will be provided, including the controversial areas surrounding decision-making and timing for adrenalectomy.

Keywords: management, medical, surgery, adrenalectomy

1. Introduction

Pheochromocytomas are rare tumours of the sympathetic nervous system that arise from the chromaffin cells of the adrenal medulla. These tumours secrete catecholamines either intermittently or continuously. Pheochromocytomas are generally unilateral, in 90% of cases, whereas bilateral disease is found more commonly in the paediatric population and associated with genetic syndromes. Right-sided adrenal tumours are more common and have a higher preponderance to cause paroxysmal hypertension compared to left-sided tumours that are generally associated with persistent hypertension. These tumours have an estimated incidence of 2–8 cases per million per year [1] and comprise less than 0.1% of the hypertensive population; however, approximately 90% of all patients with pheochromocytoma have associated hypertension [2]. Classic presentation of pheochromocytoma consists of a triad of symptoms, including headaches, diaphoresis and palpitations. The gold standard of treatment for pheochromocytoma is elective surgical resection after an appropriate, usually 1–2 weeks, course of anti-hypertensive therapy.

Pheochromocytoma multisystem crisis (PMC) was a term first described in 1988 [3]. This rare and potentially fatal entity consists of a tetrad of symptoms including haemodynamic instability and collapse, encephalopathy, hyperthermia and multi-organ failure. PMC is not synonymous with hypertensive crisis; patients with PMC typically tend to have very labile blood pressures ranging from severe hypotension to severe hypertension (e.g. 60–250 mm Hg systolic). The treatment of PMC remains controversial, as there is no consensus among clinicians regarding the appropriate timing of adrenalectomy in the specific setting of pheochromocytoma crisis. This chapter will address the clinical presentation of PMC, pathophysiology of pheochromocytoma, causes of PMC and a description of medical versus surgical treatment. Finally, the evidence regarding emergency adrenalectomy to treat PMC compared with medical management will be discussed.

2. Clinical presentation

Pheochromocytoma has been termed the 'great mimicker' because it presents in a non-specific way that may be mistaken for other clinical entities. Patients presented with the classic triad of pheochromocytoma (i.e. headaches, palpitations and diaphoresis) may initially be given the misdiagnosis of migraine headaches or psychiatric conditions such as acute anxiety or panic attacks. This clinical situation can be particularly dangerous because some medications used for treatment (i.e. β-blockers) may induce paroxysms of severe hypertension and subsequent pheochromocytoma crisis. Some clinicians advocate that in cases with anxiety and/or migraines, such patients should undergo formal screening for pheochromocytoma because the treatment of the former conditions may precipitate a crisis [4].

PMC consists of a constellation of symptoms that can also resemble other life-threatening conditions and can be difficult to diagnose if the patient is not already known for pheochromocytoma. PMC, which consists of haemodynamic instability with either severe hypotension or hypertension, labile hypertension, hyperthermia (≥40°C), encephalopathy and multi-organ failure, can be confused with other diagnoses such as septic shock, thyroid storm and malignant hyperthermia. This complex can be deleterious to every organ system, resulting from excess norepinephrine secretion causing extreme vasoconstriction, but also due to vasodilatation from excess epinephrine secretion and volume contraction, with a subsequent low-flow state. Encephalopathy may occur secondary to severe hypertension or direct effects of catecholamines on the brain. Other neurologic manifestations of PMC include cerebrovascular

http://dx.doi.org/10.5772/intechopen.69338

accidents and seizures. Cardiac complications are numerous and may include cardiomyopathy, myocarditis, myocardial ischemia and necrosis secondary to coronary vasospasm, congestive heart failure, cardiac arrhythmias and cardiogenic shock. Pulmonary manifestations include pulmonary edema and acute respiratory distress syndrome. Patients with PMC may also present with acute liver failure, acute kidney injury, disseminated intravascular coagulation, lactic acidosis, diabetic ketoacidosis and rhabdomyolysis. Gastrointestinal manifestations include paralytic ileus and intestinal ischemia secondary to vasoconstriction. Vascular complications can include peripheral thrombosis, embolism and vasospasm [5, 6].

3. Pathophysiology

Pheochromocytomas arise from the chromaffin cells of the adrenal medulla. Chromaffin cells produce catecholamines, and pheochromocytomas can produce up to 27 times the synthetic capacity of the normal adrenal medulla. This high rate of production causes accumulation of catecholamines and their metabolites, metanephrines, in the cytoplasm of the chromaffin cells, which then diffuse out of the cells into the vascular system [2]. Tumour size directly correlates with levels of catecholamine secretion with smaller tumours secreting fewer hormones than larger tumours, whereas larger tumours reported to have wider variability of hormone secretion [7]. Most pheochromocytomas produce epinephrine and norepinephrine, which both act on G-protein coupled adrenergic receptors [8].

Norepinephrine acts on α-1-adrenergic receptors that are located on smooth muscle cells within peripheral arteries and veins, causing vasoconstriction; α-2-adrenergic receptors, located on the presynaptic surface of sympathetic ganglia, cause coronary vasoconstriction and peripheral arterial dilatation; and β-1-adrenergic receptors located on cardiomyocytes, cause positive inotropic effects, as depicted in **Figure 1**. Activation of β-1-adrenergic receptors also causes increased secretion of renin, which increases the mean arterial pressure. Epinephrine primarily acts on β-1- and β-2-adrenergic receptors. Activation of β-2-adrenergic receptors leads to vasodilatation of arteries as well as increased secretion of norepinephrine by the sympathetic ganglia.

Depending on the catecholamine secretory profile of the tumour, pheochromocytomas can have different clinical manifestations. Most pheochromocytomas secrete more norepinephrine than epinephrine; however, they can secrete both hormones or secrete epinephrine alone. Severe hypertension may develop because of vasoconstriction from excess norepinephrine secretion whereas severe hypotension may result from widespread vasodilation caused by excess epinephrine secretion. Other mechanisms have been postulated to explain these changes in blood pressure. One of the explanations is that tumour necrosis may cause overwhelming tumour cell death and an abrupt cessation of catecholamine secretion, thereby leading to severe hypotension. However, it has also been postulated that tumour cell death may lead to cell lysis and subsequent massive release of catecholamines and severe hypertension. It is unclear which pathophysiologic mechanisms are responsible for the haemodynamic instability associated with PMC, but each mechanism likely contributes to the overall clinical picture.

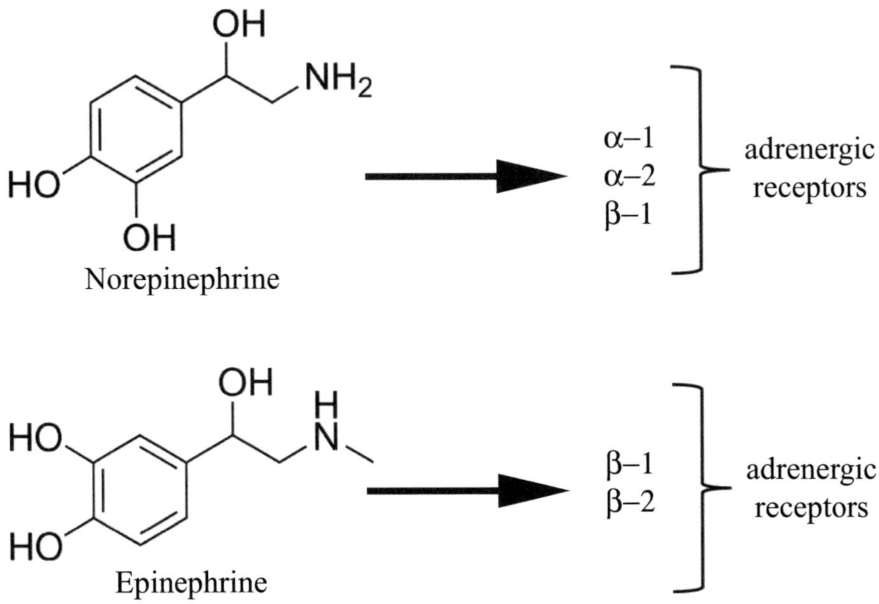

Figure 1. Illustration of catecholamine-receptor interaction.

4. Causes

Pheochromocytomas can cause sustained hypertension if there is continuous secretion of catecholamines, but can also cause paroxysmal hypertension with associated symptoms. If the paroxysm is severe, it may precipitate PMC, as reviewed in **Table 1**. PMC can occur spontaneously, if there is necrosis or haemorrhage of the tumour itself or if there is any source of external pressure on the tumour. Changes in body position, for example, even something as benign as rolling over in bed, may induce PMC [2]. Vigorous exercise, especially if it involves bending and lifting, may also precipitate PMC, as well as any kind of trauma.

PMC may also occur in the perioperative period, in the setting of adrenalectomy or any other operative indication. PMC can be triggered by certain anaesthetic agents upon induction of general anaesthesia, upon incubation, bladder catheterization, surgical skin incision, establishment of pneumoperitoneum and surgical manipulation of the tumour itself [9]. Anxiety and stress may also trigger an episode of PMC. Certain foods, such as aged cheeses, beer, wine, meats, fish, bananas and chocolate, especially those containing tyramine, have been reported to induce PMC [2].

Finally, many medications have been associated with PMC, including β-blockers, glucocorticoids, metoclopramide, various anaesthetic agents, tricyclic anti-depressants, MAO inhibitors, opiates, methyldopa, nicotine, cocaine and certain radio contrast media. The use of non-selective β-blockers causes unopposed activation of α-adrenergic receptors, thus exacerbating vasoconstriction and worsening hypertension. Glucocorticoid administration may cause PMC

Spontaneous	• Tumour necrosis • Tumour haemorrhage • Patient factors, e.g. anxiety, stress
Related to movement	• Changes in body position, e.g. rolling over in bed • Vigorous exercise • Trauma
Periprocedural/perioperative	• Induction of general anaesthesia • Incubation • Bladder catheterization • Surgical skin incision • Pneumoperitoneum • Surgical manipulation of the tumour
Medications	• β-blockers • Glucocorticoids • Metoclopramide • Anaesthetic agents: Intravenous, e.g. ketamine, atropine; inhalational, e.g. halothane, desflurane • Paralytics: succinylcholine, pancuronium • Antidepressants: Tricyclic agents, monoamine oxidase inhibitors • Methyldopa • Nicotine • Cocaine
Food	• Tyramine-containing: Aged cheeses, wine • Beer • Meats • Fish • Bananas • Chocolate
Special circumstance	• Pregnancy: Normal foetal movements, compression of the tumour during labour, increased intra-abdominal pressure during labour and delivery

Table 1. Causes of pheochromocytoma multisystem crisis.

by stimulating catecholamine release from the tumour itself and also by potentiating the effects of catecholamines at the level of the endothelial and smooth muscle cells in the peripheral vasculature [10]. Metoclopramide may cause PMC by stimulating catecholamine release by acting on serotonin type 4 receptors [11]. Any anaesthetic agent that induces catecholamine surges or histamine may precipitate PMC and may include: ketamine, which has sympathomimetic effects; succinylcholine, which can cause catecholamine surges and stimulation of autonomic ganglia, as well as possibly causing mechanical stimulation via muscle fasciculations in close proximity to the tumour; pancuronium, atropine and inhalational anaesthetics such as halothane, which is arrhythmogenic and desflurane, which is a sympathomimetic drug [9].

Special considerations should be made for pheochromocytoma in the context of pregnancy, as there may be adverse effects to both mother and foetus. PMC can be triggered by increased intra-abdominal pressure during gestation and normal labour and delivery, normal foetal movements or tumour compression during labour. PMC almost inevitably occurs with vaginal delivery, and for this reason, pregnant patients with pheochromocytoma in the antepartum period should be delivered by Caesarean section. Depending on when the diagnosis of pheochromocytoma is made, the patient should undergo laparoscopic resection in the first or second trimester, or at time of Caesarean section after delivery. Unrecognized pheochromocytomas have been associated with very high incidences of morbidity and mortality, with reported values of 40% for maternal mortality and 56% for foetal mortality [2]. While maternal catecholamines do not cross the placenta, they can cause uteroplacental insufficiency and subsequent foetal demise [2].

5. Treatment options

Medical management of pheochromocytoma is necessary prior to surgical resection. For PMC, every attempt should be made to control labile blood pressure to reduce or stop the progression of symptoms and thereby stabilize the patient. Many different classes of anti-hypertensive agents can be used to treat hypertension in pheochromocytoma preoperatively before elective adrenalectomy. Intravenous agents such as phentolamine, a parenteral, short-acting α-adrenergic blocker; nitroprusside; nitroglycerin; nicardipine, a calcium-channel blocker; atenolol or esmolol, β-adrenergic blockers and magnesium sulphate have all been shown to effectively treat hypertensive crisis. Intravenous lidocaine is also used to treat cardiac arrhythmias seen in PMC.

The first-line agents are α-adrenergic blockers, the most common of which is phenoxybenzamine, which is a non-selective blocker with a long half-life. Phenoxybenzamine decreases blood pressure, but may also increase the risk of tachycardia and decrease the risk of cardiac arrhythmias; this mechanism of action is achieved by blocking α-adrenergic receptors and not by decreasing the synthesis of catecholamines. Selective α-blockers are also used, including doxazosin and prazosin, which are as effective at treating haemodynamic instability as the non-selective α-blockers. These agents are associated with less reflex tachycardia and less post-operative hypotension than non-selective α-blockers.

Calcium channel blockers (e.g. nifedipine, verapamil or diltiazem) are better tolerated by patients than α-blockers; however, they are less effective therefore not usually a first-line choice. Angiotensin-converting enzyme inhibitors and angiotensin receptor blockers have also been used to control hypertension in pheochromocytoma, but not as first-line agents and they usually used in combination with other classes of medications to more effectively control blood pressure. Only β-adrenergic blockers are typically administered after α-blockers have been started, and they are used specifically to treat persistent tachycardia. Non-selective β-blockers should not be used in the treatment of pheochromocytoma because of their effects on β-2-adrenergic receptors, which inhibit vasodilatation and worsen hypertension. Instead, selective β-blockers should be prescribed at low doses as they act solely on β-1-adrenergic receptors, thereby decreasing heart rate. Alpha-methyl-para-tyrosine can also be used to treat hypertension in pheochromocytoma, as it interrupts the first step in the biosynthesis of catecholamines by inhibiting the enzyme tyrosine hydroxylase. However, this drug has severe adverse effects that include psychiatric disturbances, extrapyramidal symptoms, sedation and urolithiasis, and its use, therefore, is generally reserved for patients with malignant or metastatic pheochromocytoma.

Surgical resection remains the definitive treatment for pheochromocytoma. Laparoscopic transperitoneal adrenalectomy is most commonly performed; however, other operations may be used, such as the lateral retroperitoneal, posterior retroperitoneal and transthoracic surgical approaches. Successful adrenalectomy requires close communication between the surgical team and the anaesthesiology team, especially at the time of adrenal vein dissection and division, as the patient may develop profound hypotension once the vein is ligated. Tumour and adrenal gland manipulation should be minimized until after the vein is clipped. Timing of surgical resection in the context of PMC is very controversial, and there is no clear consensus among clinicians as to whether emergency adrenalectomy is indicated and/or is considered safe for PMC. The following section will review the literature pertaining to the treatment options, decision-making and outcomes in PMC.

6. Initial management: when is it appropriate to operate?

The treatment of PMC has traditionally consisted of immediate medical stabilization followed by emergent or urgent adrenalectomy. There are three treatment options in the case of PMC, including: (1) **emergent adrenalectomy**, i.e. once the diagnosis of PMC is made, the patient proceeds directly to surgery; (2) **urgent adrenalectomy**, i.e. the patient's haemodynamic status is first treated medically with a short course of α-blockade prior to adrenalectomy, usually within 7–10 days of presentation and within the same hospital admission and (3) **elective adrenalectomy**, i.e. planned surgery following initial medical stabilization and discharge from hospital. The tendency for emergency adrenalectomy was based on anecdotal evidence from published case reports suggesting that medical management alone led to poorer outcomes. In 1980, one group recommended that only brief attempts should be made to stabilize the patient's haemodynamic and that 'procrastination' prior to operative intervention would lead to 'irreversible shock, renal failure and death' [12]. In their series, two patients who presented with 'acute pheochromocytoma' both died, one in the post-operative period and one in whom the diagnosis of pheochromocytoma had not been established. Another group published a case series that included three cases of PMC [13]. One patient's hypertensive crisis was successfully controlled prior to operative intervention, however, upon development of a fever of 40°C, a septic workup was initiated and the patient became encephalopathic, leading to respiratory distress and had fatal cardiac arrhythmias while awaiting surgery. The second patient in their series presented with syncope and quickly developed multisystem organ failure despite adequate blood pressure control with multiple α- and β-blocking agents. Urgent adrenalectomy was eventually performed 4 days after hospital admission. The operation was successful, but the patient's post-operative course was prolonged and she was left with long-term sequelae of her encephalopathy, including quadriplegia and dysarthria. The third patient in the case series also presented with hypertensive crisis with rapid deterioration to multisystem organ failure, and underwent emergency adrenalectomy on the seventh day following admission for refractory multi-organ failure. Surgery was successful, and the patient's multisystem crisis resolved post-operatively.

More recently, several case reports have been published that also support urgent operative intervention in the setting of PMC. In 2008, a study described a case of PMC upon induction of general anaesthesia in the context of elective adrenalectomy for a known pheochromocytoma, despite preoperative α-blockade [14]. Surgical resection was aborted, and the patient was transferred to the authors' institution, where he remained in the intensive care unit for 6 days for aggressive medical stabilization followed by urgent adrenalectomy. The patient eventually recovered from his multisystem organ failure and discharged from the hospital 1 month later. In 2010, a reported case of PMC was described that initially presented with acute respiratory failure and encephalopathy, in which surgical resection was performed 11 days after admission because of the patient's progressive and uncontrollable medical deterioration [5]. Post-operatively, the patient's condition improved almost immediately, and the multisystem organ failure resolved except for chronic renal failure requiring long-term haemodialysis. In another case report of a patient who presented with acute heart failure with cardiogenic shock refractory to inotropic pharmacotherapy, insertion of an intra-aortic balloon pump was required, and extracorporeal membrane oxygenation (ECMO) was considered. The treating physicians, however, elected to proceed with emergent adrenalectomy. The patient's haemodynamic and respiratory status greatly improved shortly after surgery [15].

Several other authors have challenged the notion that the only viable option for the treatment of PMC is emergency adrenalectomy. Elective adrenalectomy following intensive medical stabilization has been shown in several case reports. In a 12-year-old child, with severe dilated cardiomyopathy, secondary to excess catecholamine secretion from a pheochromocytoma was treated with anti-hypertensives, specifically phenoxybenzamine and α-methyl-para-tyrosine, for 7 months prior to surgical resection [16]. Cardiac function improved moderately with medical management alone in the preoperative period and normalized completely post-operatively. Another report described two cases of PMC resulting in respiratory failure requiring incubation and ventilation, and acute kidney injury requiring continuous venovenous haemodialysis [4]. Adrenalectomy was performed at least 1 month after initial presentation, following medical stabilization and maintenance.

The case reports above describe the clinical presentation of PMC in detail, but there is very limited data regarding the perioperative management of PMC and whether it is preferable to proceed with emergency surgery with preoperative α-blockade versus medical management alone in the immediate period of crisis, followed by hospital discharge and elective adrenalectomy. Current review of the literature only reports anecdotal evidence and consequently subject to publication bias. However, a recent retrospective chart review of PMC cases at their institution as well as a literature review of all cases of PMC that underwent adrenalectomy was performed [6]. The authors reviewed medical charts from March 1993 to October 2011 of all patients who underwent adrenalectomy for a diagnosis of pheochromocytoma or paraganglionoma confirmed by pathology. They defined pheochromocytoma crisis as severe hypertension or hypotension resulting in end-organ damage, and found that 25 of 137 patients presented with crisis. None of the patients in their series underwent emergency surgery without initial α-blockade. All but one patient was stabilized with phenoxybenzamine prior to adrenalectomy. Ten patients underwent urgent adrenalectomy during the same hospital admission, whereas the other 15 patients were discharged from hospital and returned for elective adrenalectomy. There were no mortalities in either group, but the major clinical significant difference was that there was an increased use of intra-aortic balloon pumps, higher incidence of preoperative ICU admissions for crisis, higher post-operative complication rate, increased post-operative ICU admissions and longer post-operative length of stay in the urgent surgery group.

In their literature review, the authors found 97 patients who underwent adrenalectomy for PMC. In this group, they identified three different management options: emergency surgery without prior α-blockade, urgent surgery with α-blockade and medical stabilization and elective surgery post-discharge after medical therapy to initially treat the crisis. The combined data for patients undergoing elective and urgent surgery were compared to the emergency surgery group. The most striking significant difference between these groups was the mortality rate, which was found to be 18% in emergency surgery patients compared to 0% in the elective/urgent surgery patients. There were other statistically significant differences, such as increased preoperative diagnosis of pheochromocytoma in the elective/urgent patients, higher incidence of tumour haemorrhage or rupture in the emergency surgery patients, higher incidence and longer duration of preoperative α-blockade in the elective/urgent surgery patients, higher rate of laparoscopy in the elective/urgent surgery patients and increased risks of both intra-operative and post-operative complications in the emergency surgery patients.

Currently, this is the only large-scale study available regarding the management of pheochromocytoma crisis. Based on their experience from their own institutions, it appears feasible and safe to attempt medical therapy and elective adrenalectomy if the patient can be discharged safely from hospital, as outcomes are better for patients undergoing elective compared to urgent surgical resection during the same admission. From the data available in the literature, it is quite clear that emergency adrenalectomy without adequate preoperative α-blockade is associated with high morbidity and mortality in the treatment of PMC. It is therefore recommended to offer urgent adrenalectomy in those patients who are able to partially recover under intensive medical management, while elective adrenalectomy can be reserved for patients who fully recover with medical management and who can safely be discharged from the hospital. Ideally, adrenalectomy should be planned within 4–6 weeks following discharge. This study is limited in that it is a retrospective review, but since PMC is such a rare clinical entity, it would be very unlikely that a prospective, randomized study could ever be carried out [6]. Nevertheless, it seems clear that emergency adrenalectomy should be discouraged as an initial treatment of PMC and that medical therapy and eventual urgent or elective surgery should be the preferred management if the patient's condition allows it. A flow diagram for decision-making in patients with pheochromocytoma crisis is shown in **Figure 2**.

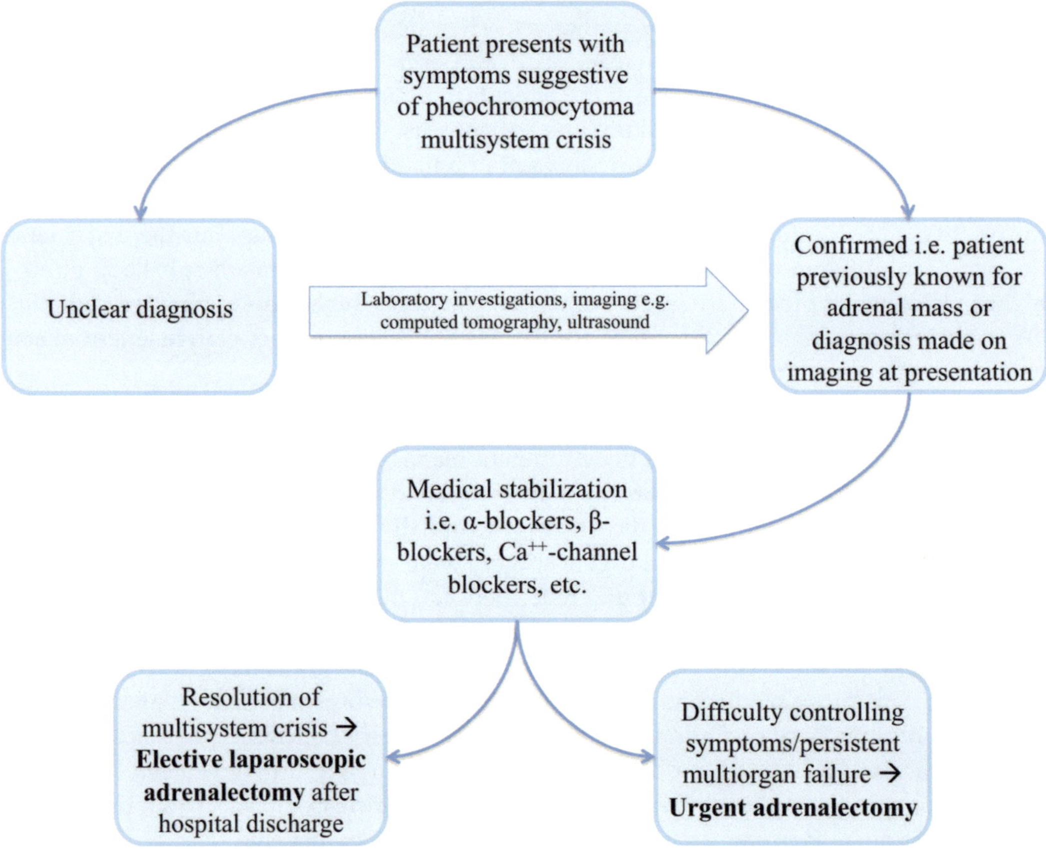

Figure 2. Decision-making flow chart for patients presenting with PMC.

7. Conclusion

There has been a paradigm shift in the surgical management of PMC, from performing emergency adrenalectomy immediately after the diagnosis to now favouring medical stabilization followed by elective adrenalectomy in more controlled and ideal situation, but allowing for urgent adrenalectomy in the same hospital admission if necessary. There are currently no guidelines available or Level 1 evidence to support this change in practice, and randomized studies would be impractical to perform due to the rare presentation of this clinical entity.

Further retrospective studies with larger sample sizes may be helpful in discerning the clinical outcomes of different management strategies and making a stronger recommendation for the preferred treatment of PMC.

Author details

Tanya Castelino and Elliot Mitmaker*

*Address all correspondence to: elliot.mitmaker@mcgill.ca

McGill University Health Centre, Montreal, Canada

References

[1] Reisch N, et al. Pheochromocytoma: presentation, diagnosis and treatment. Journal of Hypertension. 2006;**24**(12): 2331–2339

[2] Gardner D, Shoback D, editors. Greenspan's Basic & Clinical Endocrinology. 9th ed. China: The McGraw-Hill Companies, Inc.; 2011

[3] Newell K, et al. Pheochromocytoma crisis. American Journal of Hypertension. 1988;**1** (3 Pt 3):189s-191s

[4] Kolhe N. et al. Hypertension due to phaeochromocytoma – An unusual cause of multiorgan failure. Nephrology Dialysis Transplantation. 2001;**16**(10):2100–2104

[5] Uchida N, et al. Pheochromocytoma multisystem crisis successfully treated by emergency surgery: Report of a case. Surgery Today. 2010;**40**(10):990–996

[6] Scholten A, et al. Pheochromocytoma crisis is not a surgical emergency. Journal of Clinical Endocrinology and Metabolism. 2013;**98**(2):581–591

[7] Guerrero MA, et al. Clinical spectrum of pheochromocytoma. Journal of the American College of Surgeons. 2009;**209**(6): 727–732

[8] Zuber SM, Kantorovich V, Pacak K. Hypertension in pheochromocytoma: Characteristics and treatment. Endocrinology and Metabolism Clinics of North America. 2011;**40**(2):295–311

[9] Ramakrishna H. Pheochromocytoma resection: Current concepts in anesthetic management. Journal of Anaesthesiology, Clinical Pharmacology. 2015;**31**(3):317–323

[10] Rosas AL, et al. Pheochromocytoma crisis induced by glucocorticoids: A report of four cases and review of the literature. European Journal of Endocrinology. 2008;**158**(3):423–429

[11] Guillemot J, et al. Metoclopramide stimulates catecholamine- and granin-derived peptide secretion from pheochromocytoma cells through activation of serotonin type 4 (5-HT4) receptors. Endocrine-Related Cancer. 2009;**16**(1):281–290

[12] Freier DT, Eckhauser FE, Harrison TS. Pheochromocytoma. A persistently problematic and still potentially lethal disease. Archives of Surgery. 1980;**115**(4):388–391

[13] Newell KA, et al. Pheochromocytoma multisystem crisis. A surgical emergency. Archives of Surgery. 1988;**123**(8):956–959

[14] Solorzano CC, Parks J, Prinz RA. Pheochromocytoma presenting with multiple organ failure. American Journal of Surgery. 2008;**74**(11):1119–1121

[15] Salinas CL, et al. Emergency adrenalectomy due to acute heart failure secondary to complicated pheochromocytoma: a case report. World Journal of Surgical Oncology. 2011;**9**:49

[16] Imperato-McGinley J, et al. Reversibility of catecholamine-induced dilated cardiomyopathy in a child with a pheochromocytoma. New England Journal of Medicine. 1987;**316**(13):793–797

Chapter 7

Current Approaches in the Minimally Invasive Surgical Treatment of Adrenal Tumors

Pasquale Cianci, Alberto Fersini, Nicola Tartaglia,
Sabino Capuzzolo, Libero Luca Giambavicchio,
Antonio Ambrosi and Vincenzo Neri

Additional information is available at the end of the chapter

http://dx.doi.org/10.5772/intechopen.69419

Abstract

The use of imaging modalities and minimally invasive surgery plays an important role in the current management of adrenal tumors. Ultrasonography frequently allows for the incidental diagnosis of adrenal masses. The most frequent adrenal pathologies encountered are hypercortisolism (Cushing's syndrome), primary hyperaldosteronism (Conn's syndrome), and pheochromocytomas. Clinical presentation of these adrenal tumors can often be non-specific, or such lesions may present as "incidentalomas" in patients who undergo imaging for clinical reasons unrelated to the adrenal glands. Adrenal malignancy is suggested by morphologic characteristics found on imaging studies: increased size, irregular borders, local invasion, and large necrotic areas. The risk of malignancy increases for larger adrenal masses. Minimally invasive surgery has become the initial choice for the treatment of adrenal tumors with retroperitoneal and transperitoneal approaches. This chapter describes the surgical indications and compares the various minimally invasive surgical approaches for the therapeutic management of adrenal masses.

Keywords: minimally invasive adrenalectomy, laparoscopic adrenalectomy, transperitoneal adrenalectomy, robotic adrenalectomy, NOTES

1. Introduction

Two main factors that have advanced the clinical management of adrenal tumors in the past 20 years include the technologic progress and widespread use of imaging studies such as ultrasonography (US), computed tomography (CT), magnetic resonance imaging (MRI), and the advent and implementation of minimally invasive surgery. In many parts of the world, US frequently allows for the incidental diagnosis of adrenal tumors. The prevalence of adrenal "incidentalomas" in autopsy series reaches 8%, whereas in imaging studies, incidentalomas occur in 4% of patients. The prevalence of adrenal incidentalomas may increase because of the improvement and widespread use of abdominal imaging [1, 2]. Minimally invasive adrenalectomy has become the initial treatment of benign adrenal tumors with transperitoneal and retroperitoneal approaches. This chapter evaluates the surgical indications and compares the various minimally invasive approaches and outcomes in the surgical management of adrenal masses.

2. Adrenal pathology

The adrenal gland encompasses two distinct tissue zones with different functional activities. The adrenal medulla, derived from neuroectodermal cells, produces catecholamines, such as epinephrine and metanephrine. The adrenal cortex, derived from mesenchymal cells, is formed by three concentric zones: the granulosa that secretes aldosterone, the fasciculata that secretes cortisol, and the inner reticularis that secretes androgens. The most frequent clinical presentations of adrenal disease are related to the hypersecretion of these adrenal hormones.

2.1. Hypercortisolism

High levels of plasma glucocorticoids or hypercortisolism result in the classic symptoms and clinical features associated with Cushing's syndrome [3]. Clinical features suggestive of hypercortisolism include central obesity, proximal myopathy, spontaneous bruising, facial plethora, wide purplish striae (>1 cm), hypokalemia, and osteoporosis. Clinical presentation of hypercortisolism can be assessed in patients by following changes in appearance from serial photographs. Cushing's syndrome may be differentiated from ACTH-dependent (e.g., pituitary adenoma, ectopic ACTH secretion), and ACTH-independent (e.g., adrenal adenoma, adrenal carcinoma, adrenal hyperplasia). ACTH-independent Cushing's syndrome due to adrenal adenoma or carcinoma can be surgically treated with adrenalectomy.

2.2. Primary hyperaldosteronism

The most common type of primary hyperaldosteronism is caused by aldosterone-producing adenomas, and less frequently, bilateral idiopathic adrenal hyperplasia. Solitary adrenal adenomas associated with primary hyperaldosteronism are usually <2cm in size [4]. Clinically characterized by symptoms of moderate or severe hypertension and hypokalemia, patients with primary hyperaldosteronism may also have polyuria, nocturia, polydipsia, and paraesthesias. Hypertension is usually refractory to conventional antihypertensive agents. The major diagnostic challenge is distinguishing between aldosterone-producing adenomas and idiopathic hyperaldosteronism. In the former, patients have severe hypertension, higher likelihood of hypokalemia, decrease or little (<30%) increase of serum aldosterone level in upright posture test, and an adrenal mass (>1 cm) on CT. In idiopathic hyperaldosteronism, hypertension is less severe and hypokalemia less frequent. The increase of serum aldosterone level reaches >30% with upright posture test, and CT usually shows bilateral thickening of adrenal glands. For unilateral aldosterone-producing adenomas (localized lesions by imaging), surgical resection should be performed, whereas medical treatment using eplerenone (steroid-based anti-mineralocorticoid), spironolactone, and triamterene should be reserved for patients with idiopathic hyperaldosteronism.

2.3. Pheochromocytoma

Pheochromocytomas are chromaffin cell tumors, and their clinical presentation is associated with excess catecholamine production. Such adrenal tumors are usually sporadic and benign. Paragangliomas or extra-adrenal pheochromocytomas are usually located (75%) in para-aortic areas (e.g., organ of Zuckerkandl) or less frequently within the bladder, thorax, or neck. The majority of pheochromocytomas are unilateral, whereas bilateral lesions occur in 5–10% of cases and frequently as part of a familial syndrome. Pheochromocytomas can be associated with MEN2A and MEN2B syndromes, von Recklinghausen's disease, and tuberous sclerosis. Pheochromocytomas are malignant in 10% of cases with higher prevalence in ectopic locations. For malignancy, there are no clinical, laboratory, or imaging criteria. Only larger adrenal size (generally >4–5 cm) is useful to predict malignancy. Diagnostic certainty of malignant lesions is based on the presence of metastasis, not histologic features of the tumor. Clinical presentation of pheochromocytomas can encompass paroxysmal (48%), and persistent hypertension (29%) in patients. Only 10% of patients present with normotensive blood pressure. Other clinical manifestations include headaches, palpitations, diaphoresis, orthostatic hypotension, weight loss, dyspnea, polyuria, and polydipsia [5].

Plasma-free metanephrines that include total-free normetanephrines and metanephrines have 99 and 97% sensitivity, respectively. If plasma metanephrine levels are more than three or four times the upper limit of normal, specificity reaches 100% for pheochromocytomas. CT and MRI studies can detect pheochromocytomas that are ≥2 cm, and those cystic lesions with areas of necrosis. If CT or MRI does not localize the adrenal tumor, functional imaging with meta-iodobenzylguanidine (MIBG) can be useful.

Minimally invasive adrenalectomy (e.g., laparoscopic transperitoneal approach) is the initial surgical treatment of choice for benign pheochromocytomas. Adequate medical preparation before surgical resection is essential for operative success.

2.4. Incidentalomas

Adrenal incidentalomas are usually benign adrenal masses (≥1 cm) discovered "incidentally" on imaging studies conducted for other reasons not related to the adrenal glands. Current widespread use of imaging studies has led to increased discovery of incidental adrenal tumors in patients. Prevalence of incidentalomas reaches 8% in autopsy series and 4–6% in imaging studies [1, 2]. The definition of adrenal incidentaloma should be excluded in patients with known malignant disease and in patients with clinical evidence of adrenal disease. The initial evaluation of adrenal incidentalomas should define benignity or malignancy, and underlying hormonal hyperactivity. Adrenal incidentalomas are hormonally hyperactive in 35% of cases. All patients with an incidental adrenal tumor should undergo hormonal evaluation for hypercortisolism, primary hyperaldosteronism, and pheochromocytoma. Other functional evaluation (e.g., androgen hypersecretion) can also be determined by clinical manifestation. Surgical indication for non-functional adrenal incidentalomas is principally guided by tumor size. Surgical excision is recommended for adrenal tumors >4 cm since most of the adrenocortical carcinomas (ACC) are usually large [6].

2.5. Adrenal malignancy

Primary adrenal malignancies are rare and encompass adrenocortical carcinoma (ACC) and malignant pheochromocytoma. ACC comprises 0.2% of all cancers, and these tumors can secrete excess cortisol, aldosterone, and androgens [19, 20]. Pheochromocytomas can be sporadic, hereditary, or part of MEN2A or MEN2B syndrome. Furthermore, the incidence of malignant pheochromocytoma ranges from 5 to 26% [21]. The diagnosis of malignant pheochromocytoma by imaging is based on local invasion and distal metastasis; the histologic diagnosis is frequently indeterminate due to uncertain criteria.

Assessment for adrenal malignancy is based on the size on imaging studies. Larger adrenal masses are associated with increased risk for malignancy. More specifically, incidental, non-functioning adrenal masses that measure ≥4 cm have an increased rate of malignancy and should be surgically removed. Furthermore, some reports suggest that imaging studies can delineate malignant from benign adrenal lesions. Non-contrast CT attenuation coefficient in Hounsfield units (HU) of an adrenal mass revealing densitometry <10 HU demonstrates high fat composition and increases the likelihood of a benign adenoma. CT sensitivity and specificity are 71 and 98%, respectively. Unfortunately, several adrenal adenomas (30%) are lipid-poor, and unenhanced CT is not indicative [7, 8].

The risk of malignancy is very high for larger adrenal tumors with a size threshold of 4 cm having a sensitivity of 96% and specificity of 52% for cancer. An adrenal tumor size threshold of 6 cm has a sensitivity of 90% and specificity of 80% for malignancy [9]. Adrenal tumor size not only suggests malignancy risk but also a criterion of reference for the choice surgical approach. Adrenal malignancy is also suggested by morphologic characteristics by imaging studies including irregular border, local invasion, large necrotic areas and infiltration of the tumor into the periadrenal fat [9]. Other malignant adrenal lesions are metastases from lung, breast, and other non-adrenal cancers. Removal of such adrenal masses does not commonly occur as the only site of metastatic disease [10, 11].

Fine-needle aspiration of adrenal masses is not an initial diagnostic test. It is primarily useful in cases of suspected metastatic lesions. Most adrenal lesions, within the realm of surgical treatment, are unilateral benign tumors including pheochromocytomas, adrenocortical adenomas, and adrenal incidentalomas. Other less common surgical indications include adrenal cysts, ganglioneuromas, myelolipomas, androgen-secreting tumors, and bilateral lesions such as macronodular adrenal hyperplasia.

3. Indication for adrenalectomy

The size threshold of benign and functional adrenal tumors for laparoscopic adrenalectomy has traditionally ranged from 8 to 9 cm. Nevertheless, the size limit of adrenal masses for laparoscopic resection has incrementally increased following the improvement in surgical skills and technologies. Some limitation criteria for laparoscopic removal such as size >9 cm, and preoperative radiologic evidence of and/or intraoperative local infiltration of periadrenal tissue may be useful in patient selection.

A remaining controversial issue is the laparoscopic resection of highly suspicious or malignant adrenal masses. In the opinion of the authors, well-defined local invasiveness is essential for determining the suitability for laparoscopic adrenalectomy [12–18]. Recent data from the literature confirm that laparoscopic adrenalectomy can replicate open surgical oncologic resection of ACC, showing comparable survival and recurrence rates. The most important contraindication for the minimally invasive adrenalectomy is local infiltration of periadrenal tissue determined by preoperative imaging and intraoperative inspection.

Adrenal metastases may come from primary tumors of lung, breast, stomach, and kidney. Detection of metastasis has increased with the widespread use of imaging studies for cancer surveillance. If solitary metastatic lesions are limited within the capsule of the adrenal gland, adrenalectomy can be performed [22]. Laparoscopic adrenalectomy can also be performed for high-risk lesions for malignancy, but general experience is limited, and oncologic effectiveness of minimally invasive approaches remains uncertain in this setting [12, 17, 18, 23–28].

When malignant adrenal tumors, primary or metastatic, are removed laparoscopically, surgical oncologic principles must be followed: low likelihood for conversion, complete removal with the slightest manipulation and without fragmentation of periadrenal tissues. If required, the conversion to an open procedure must be performed very early, before the advanced dissection of the operative site and possible fragmentation of periadrenal fat or tumor capsule. Recent data from the literature confirm that laparoscopic adrenalectomy is safe and effective for malignant adrenal tumors. In some studies, outcome results with regard to peritoneal carcinomatosis, positive resection margins, and time to recurrence showed no statistically significant differences between open and laparoscopic approaches [12, 28–33]. In other studies with regard to ACC, oncologic outcomes of laparoscopic adrenalectomy were not comparable to open adrenalectomy [17, 34, 35].

4. Minimally invasive surgery for adrenal tumors

The surgical approach to the adrenal glands has evolved considerably from the description of the first laparoscopic adrenalectomy by Gagner et al. [36]. This minimally invasive surgical approach has established itself as the "gold standard" for the surgical treatment of most adrenal lesions. The advantages in performing laparoscopic adrenalectomy include reduced hospital stay, fewer complications, and better aesthetic results. Traditional open adrenalectomy is still reserved for malignant or larger adrenal tumors [37, 38]. Regardless of approach, the key to successful adrenalectomy remains the same: proper patient selection for surgery, solid understanding of adrenal pathophysiology, and a thorough knowledge of adrenal anatomy. Over the last two decades, many minimally invasive techniques have been introduced including the lateral transabdominal (LT), retroperitoneal (RE), anterior transabdominal (AT), hand-assisted (HA), thoracoscopic transdiaphragmatic (TT) approaches, and natural orifice transluminal endoscopic surgery (NOTES). With the advent of robotic surgery, its integration into adrenal surgery has made it feasible to offer an alternative to patients requiring surgical treatment of adrenal disorders.

The most frequently performed laparoscopic approach is LT (79%), followed by RE (32%) and AT access (14%) [39]. These different laparoscopic approaches are determined by the surgeon's skill set. Laparoscopic LT adrenalectomy is the most popular procedure as it allows for wide exposure of the retroperitoneal space and takes advantage of mobilization of organs due to gravity in both left and right lateral positions: spleen, pancreas or liver. Using laparoscopic LT access, there are no major differences between the right and left adrenalectomy except for longer operative time for left adrenal glands [40]. Open adrenalectomy consists of transabdominal or retroperitoneal approaches that can be mimicked by minimally invasive surgery for adrenal resection.

4.1. Transabdominal approach

4.1.1. Lateral

Under general anesthesia, the patient is positioned with left lateral side down for right adrenalectomy and the right lateral side down for left adrenalectomy. Pneumoperitoneum is induced through a Veress needle inserted in the flank or through a laparoscopic trocar (**Figure 1**–port **B**) with CO_2 pressure regulated at 12 mmHg for the whole procedure; a 0°/30° laparoscope is introduced through this port. Three other 10 mm (**Figure 1** ports **A-C-D**) ports are inserted for the introduction of atraumatic graspers, hook, retractors, an instrument with peanut swab, and scissors.

For left adrenalectomy, the first step of intervention is dissection and mobilization of pancreaticosplenic bloc by the division of the splenorenal ligament. The lateral position of the patient allows for better mobilization of the spleen and pancreatic tail (**Figure 2**). In some patients, the division of phrenocolic ligament for mobilization of the left colonic flexure is useful. This mobilization allows for the exposure of the left adrenal gland that involves dissection into the retroperitoneal fat above the left kidney. Most important is the careful dissection and ligation of the left adrenal vein, usually by clips, that runs directly into a left renal vein.

For right adrenalectomy, the retroperitoneal space can be entered with incision of posterior peritoneum along the inferior visceral surface of the liver and right triangular ligament. Upper retraction of the liver to expose the surface and superior pole of the right adrenal gland is useful. Most important is the identification and exposure of the inferior vena cava (IVC). The right adrenal gland is partially retrocaval, and a very short adrenal vein runs directly into the IVC. The right adrenal vein should be carefully identified, clipped, and divided (**Figure 3**). The right adrenal gland can be dissected free from the retroperitoneal fat, hemostasis is checked, and the adrenal bed is irrigated. The specimen is placed in a plastic bag and extracted through the anterior trocar.

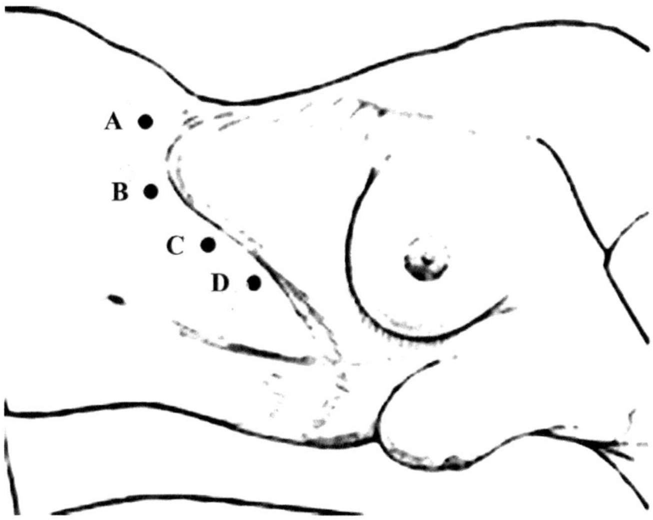

Figure 1. Trocar access in the lateral transabdominal approach.

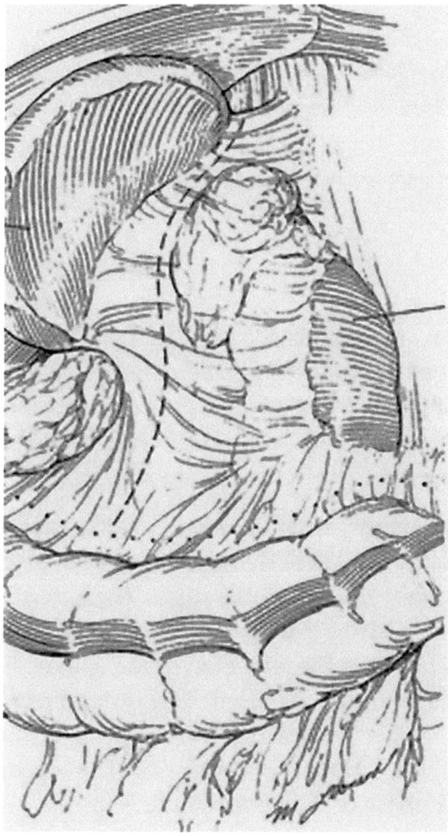

Figure 2. Laparoscopic exposure of left adrenal gland: mobilization of the spleen and tail of the pancreas and dissection of left colonic flexure.

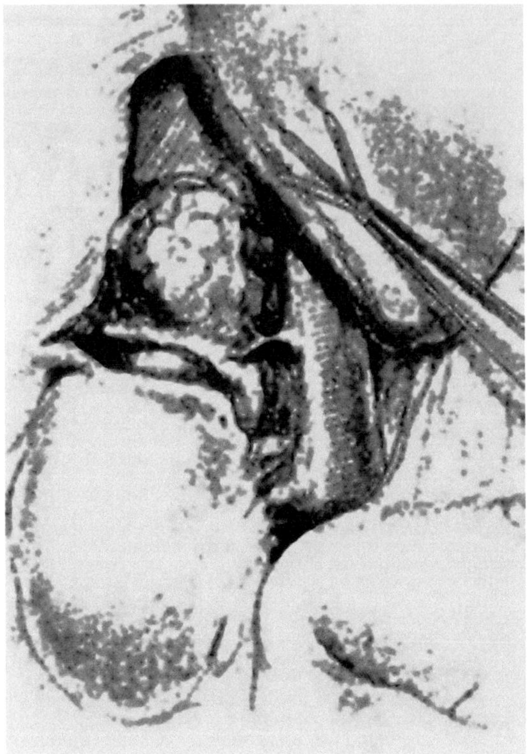

Figure 3. Laparoscopic exposure of right adrenal gland: mobilization of the liver, identification of short right adrenal vein–partial retrocaval position of the right adrenal gland.

4.1.2. Anterior

The anterior transabdominal approach is a less preferred initial choice for laparoscopic adrenalectomy [41, 42]. Under general anesthesia, the patient is placed on the operative table in the supine position with containment devices on both sides to allow for table tilting laterally, if required. Pneumoperitoneum is induced with a Veress needle at the umbilicus, or with an open technique based on surgeon preference or previous surgery.

For left adrenalectomy, four trocars are employed in the following positions: above the umbilicus, in the subxiphoid position, along with the left midclavicular line at the umbilicus level, and in the left flank region along the midaxillary line. The anterior transabdominal approach does not allow for mobilization by the gravity of the spleen and pancreatic tail. Consequently, wide dissection and mobilization of the left colon to the splenic flexure and division of splenocolic and phrenocolic ligaments are required. Exposure of the retroperitoneum allows for identification of the superior pole of left kidney and surface of the adrenal gland, which can be dissected and mobilized into retroperitoneal fat. The left adrenal vein should be identified and clipped during the first phase of the dissection [43].

For right adrenalectomy, trocar position is similar to left adrenalectomy, but on the opposite side. After separation of omental adhesions, the peritoneal reflection along the lateral side of the inferior vena cava is exposed. The incision is extended transversely to the peritoneum overlying the posterior margin of the liver. This dissection permits transverse identification of the short right adrenal vein directly entering the IVC. Liver retraction allows the surgeon to gain exposure of the upper portion of the right adrenal gland. After identification and careful dissection, the right adrenal vein is ligated with titanium clips and divided. The right adrenal gland is mobilized by blunt dissection and electrocautery until completely free. The adrenal gland is then placed into a specimen retrieval bag for removal through any of the port sites [43].

4.2. Retroperitoneal approach

Although transperitoneal techniques remain more popular and widely used, the retroperitoneal approach has several distinct advantages that make it an attractive alternative for surgical removal of adrenal tumors [41]. The retroperitoneal approach for adrenalectomy is the second most common surgical technique utilized. Some authors report the advantage of a more direct route to the adrenal gland without interference from intra-abdominal organs using the retroperitoneal approach. Furthermore, shorter operative times and hospital stay with fewer postoperative fluid collections have been reported with this technique [37, 41, 44–48]. The major difficulties associated with the retroperitoneal approach are restricted operative space and difficult detection of anatomical landmarks that may cause longer operative times and increased carbon dioxide absorption [44, 49–51].

4.2.1. Lateral

The patient is in full flank position with the operating table flexed to open the space between the iliac crest and costal margin. The procedure starts with the open insertion of a balloon trocar in the middle axillary line 3 cm above the iliac crest. After retroperitoneal dilation using a balloon, a 10 mm trocar is inserted for a 30 degree 10 mm laparoscope, and then, carbon dioxide is insufflated to generate a pneumoretroperitoneum pressure of 15 mmHg. Three other trocars are placed above the first: along the anterior axillary line, along with the lateral border of sacrospinalis muscle, and below the costal margin always along the anterior axillary line. An optional fifth port may be necessary in order to retract the liver or in cases where the peritoneum has been lacerated.

For left adrenalectomy, dissection begins along the lateral border of psoas muscle to medial border left kidney, where the left kidney is retracted upward and anteriorly. The renal hilum is isolated to identify the left renal vein and medial border of the left adrenal gland. The left adrenal vein is located at the inferomedial left adrenal gland in conjunction with the left renal vein. After identification, the left adrenal vein is ligated between clips. The adrenal gland is mobilized and separated from the left kidney, and the superior and inferior phrenic vessels are controlled with an ultrasonic coagulation instrument or bipolar cautery. The left adrenal gland is placed into a sterile plastic bag and extracted from a primary port.

For right adrenalectomy, dissection of right adrenal gland follows the same principles described for left adrenal gland dissection. The psoas muscle is an important key anatomical landmark. After identification of right kidney and right adrenal gland, careful dissection to the IVC located at the medial part of psoas muscle is performed. The right adrenal vein is identified in conjunction to the IVC, clipped, and divided. After complete excision of the right adrenal gland, the specimen is placed into a sterile plastic bag and extracted from a primary port. The trocars are removed and port sites sutured closed.

4.2.2. Posterior

The patient may be placed in the prone or jack-knife position, and this is valid for both sides. Access to the retroperitoneum begins with the insertion of a balloon trocar to 2.5 cm lateral to the tip of 12th rib and insufflated [52]. Through the balloon trocar, a laparoscope is inserted to evaluate the retroperitoneal space, and the balloon trocar is then replaced with another 10 mm trocar. CO_2 is injected at 12–20 mm Hg pressure to sustain an adequate retroperitoneal space. A second trocar is inserted under the edge of the 12th rib, the 3rd at the 11th and last at the 9th and 10th ribs. An atraumatic retractor is introduced through the inferior trocar to retract the kidney downwards and fatty tissue. Mobilization of the upper renal pole will allow visualization of the adrenal gland. A retractor inserted into the medial or lateral trocar controls the upper pole of the kidney. The adrenal gland is mobilized medially and then caudally. Between the diaphragmatic branch and adrenal gland, the arteries pass posterior to the vena cava. These vessels may be ligated by electrocautery or by clips. Dissecting the right adrenal gland superiorly will expose the vena cava posteriorly and the short adrenal vein postero-lateral that can be cleared by 1 cm and divided between clips. Continued lateral and cranial dissection will completely mobilize the right adrenal gland. The left adrenal vein is isolated in the area between the left adrenal gland and diaphragmatic branch, which is medial to the upper pole of the left kidney. The dissection of the adrenal gland continues medially, laterally and then cranially, and it will remain raised in relation only to the left renal vein. Delicate dissection with instruments is necessary to avoid damaging of the adrenal capsule.

4.3. Hand-assisted approach

The hand-assisted technique is a hybrid between the open and laparoscopic approach. For some, this technique is useful for large tumor removal with reduced surgical time [53]. For left adrenalectomy, the patient is placed in the supine position with legs separated, and two ports are inserted into the left subcostal region, and the camera port is inserted level with and lateral to the umbilicus. In the case of right adrenalectomy, two ports are placed in the right upper quadrant and another for the laparoscope that is introduced through umbilical access. The surgeon stands on the right side of the patient, and the camera operator assistant stands between the patient's legs and a second assistant retracts and assists with dissection via the remaining port sites. After the establishment of pneumoperitoneum, a midline incision is made for the placement of the HandPort for the left side, and for the right side, a right subcostal oblique incision. The size of the incision for the HandPort must be proportional to the surgeon's glove size. The HandPort base retractor is then inflated, and the surgeon connects the HandPort sleeve by initially placing the bracelet around his wrist. A second glove is then placed over the bracelet, and the back of the hand is lubricated with sterile gel. The operator's arm slides inside the sleeve of the hand port, the ring is fixed inside the abdominal incision and the basic retractor on the skin edge. The latter is inflated and the sleeve rewound and trapped in the basic retractor. Once the system is sealed, the pneumoperitoneum can be reestablished. At this point, the operator's hand can be inserted into the abdomen. To the right side, the approach is anterior, where the duodenum is mobilized, and the retroperitoneal fascia is dissected to the upper renal pole. By visualization and palpation, the surgeon begins gland dissection by isolating for the short right adrenal vein and dividing it between clips. The dissection can be performed with a combination of forceps diathermy, clips, and/or the harmonic scalpel. The left side is also performed through an anterior approach. After entering through the omentum and raising the stomach, a retroperitoneal incision along the lower edge of the body and tail of the pancreas is made. After dissection of retroperitoneal adhesions, the distal pancreas is lifted to show the left renal vein, left adrenal gland, and its central vein. The gland is dissected free from its surrounding structures, and the left adrenal vein is divided between clips [54].

4.4. Thoracoscopic transdiaphragmatic approach

The first clinical thoracoscopic adrenal biopsy was described in 1993 for non-small cell lung cancer (NSCLC) metastasis to the adrenal glands. Since then, successive experiments have described left adrenalectomy in swine models. In 2001, the access technique on four human cadavers was perfected and then performed in three patients with primary adrenal tumors and later expanded to right adrenalectomy. Transdiaphragmatic adrenalectomy was accomplished in all three cases without complication. This technique was performed after double lumen endotracheal intubation without pneumoinsufflation, and the patient was placed in the prone position. A total of four ports were used in the transthoracic approaches [55–57]. The diaphragm was incised under thoracoscope vision and then entered through the retroperitoneal space to identify the adrenal gland. The adrenal vasculature was controlled, and complete mobilization of adrenal gland was performed. The specimen was entrapped and retrieved through a thoracic port. The diaphragm was suture repaired with intracorporeal knot tying, and a chest tube was placed. Conditions that may preclude this approach include cardiopulmonary diseases and previous thoracic surgery.

4.5. Natural orifice transluminal endoscopic surgery (NOTES)

Since the first transvaginal cholecystectomy performed by Marescaux et al. 30 years ago, these procedures are performed to achieve less invasiveness during surgery [58]. Natural orifice transluminal endoscopic surgery (NOTES) is a technique that allows entry into the peritoneal cavity through transgastric or transvaginal or transcolonic access to avoid surgical scars.

Currently, NOTES has been employed on porcine and cadaveric models. Right and left adrenalectomies with a transvaginal retroperitoneal approach in a porcine model by a 1 cm posterolateral colpotomy have been performed and described [59]. The retroperitoneal tunnel is created using carbon dioxide. Dissection by movement of gastroscope up to the superior pole of kidney allows access to the adrenal gland. The vascular pedicle is identified and controlled by clips or endloop. The authors concluded that this access is also possible in human cadavers.

Zou and colleagues reportedly treated 11 consecutive women for adrenal diseases with NOTES, but with assisted-laparoscopy [60]. Under general anesthesia, patients were placed in the lithotomy position with the affected side elevated at 30°. A 5-mm trocar and a 10-mm trocar were inserted in the umbilical edge for conventional operating apparatus, and a 10-mm trocar was inserted in the posterior vaginal fornix for a conventional 30° laparoscope. Carbon dioxide pneumoperitoneum was achieved by Veress needle, and dissection was performed according to standard laparoscopic adrenalectomy with conventional operating apparatus placed in the abdomen under direct vision achieved by a conventional 30° laparoscope placed through a vaginal trocar. The dissection and mobilization of left colonic flexure for left adrenalectomy and right colonic flexure for right adrenalectomy should be performed. Similar to traditional approaches, the adrenal gland is mobilized and the vascular supply ligated. The specimen is then removed through the posterior vaginal fornix. Recent data from the literature suggest that this combined technique is feasible and effective. With ongoing development of technique and instruments, it may be an alternative technique for the treatment of some women with adrenal tumors because of its improved cosmetic results. For NOTES, further clinical studies and more practiced surgical skills are needed.

4.5.1. Robotic adrenalectomy

Although the benefits of laparoscopic adrenalectomy are well known, its drawbacks include the two-dimensional view, unstable camera platform, poor ergonomics, and rigid instrumentation. Subsequently, robotic technology has been recently introduced to join the armamentarium of minimally invasive adrenal surgery with capabilities of three-dimensional view, wristed instrument, and a stable camera platform [61]. Since the first fully robotic adrenalectomy in 2002, many studies have shown the safety and efficacy of robotic adrenalectomy (RA) [62, 63]. Transperitoneal and retroperitoneal RA approaches demonstrating the efficacy of both techniques have been described in several reports [64, 65]. Current drawbacks, however, associated with RA include its cost, technical difficulty, need of advanced training and a team with the technical expertise to ensure operative success [66–68]. It is still controversial as to whether the RA should be performed by the transperitoneal or retroperitoneal approach. Several surgeons prefer the retroperitoneal technique in patients with tumors < 6 cm in size [69]. Although it necessitates previous experience with the transperitoneal approach, the retroperitoneal approach is preferred in patients with abdominal scarring and adhesions.

Right robotic adrenalectomy is performed with the patient in the left lateral decubitus position. The table is flexed at the level of the kidneys. Trocar position and surgical steps are comparable to traditional transabdominal lateral laparoscopic adrenalectomy. The triangular liver ligament is divided as cranially as possible to release the liver. Access to retroperitoneum and right adrenal gland is obtained by incision of the posterior peritoneum along the posterior border of visceral surface of the liver with detection of the IVC. After the duodenum is kocherized, the lateral border of the IVC and right renal vein is identified. Dissecting cranially along the lateral border of the IVC, the right adrenal vein is encountered, dissected, and clipped. The right adrenal gland with any associated pathology is then progressively dissected off of the superior pole of the kidney and retroperitoneum in a circumferential manner with electrocautery. After checking for hemostasis by lowering the pneumoperitoneum, a laparoscopic entrapment sac is introduced by the assistant, and the specimen is placed into the sac. After undocking the robot, the bagged specimen is extracted through the accessory port.

Left robotic adrenalectomy is performed with the patient in the right lateral decubitus position. After the placement of the trocars in a conventional way according to the transabdominal lateral approach, the splenorenal ligament is transected. Mobilization of the spleen and pancreatic tail, made easier by gravity, allows for dissection of the left adrenal gland in the retroperitoneal fat, and identification and hemostasis of the left adrenal vein. The subsequent phases of circumferential dissection of the left adrenal gland, specimen retrieval with the closing of port-sites are identical to that described for right robotic adrenalectomy.

Comparison between laparoscopic and robotic adrenalectomy outcomes is similar including operative time, postoperative complications, hospital stay, and conversion rate [70]. In the future, RA will likely assume an increased role in the management of surgical disease. Research teams are dedicated to the development of robotic systems with greater intelligence and instruments with expanded capabilities, and it is essential that surgeons continue to evaluate these new technologies.

5. Authors' institutional experience

The surgical experience from the authors' institution that examines the outcomes of laparoscopic transperitoneal adrenalectomy is presented. Laparoscopic adrenalectomy has become the procedure of choice for most adrenal pathologies with multiple studies demonstrating significant benefits of this minimally invasive surgical approach compared to open adrenalectomy in terms of reduced operative morbidity, blood loss, analgesic requirements, shorter hospital stay, and earlier return to normal activity.

Over a 10-year period (2006–2015), the authors treated 76 patients with adrenal lesions. The laparoscopic transperitoneal approach was performed in 67 patients; open procedures were chosen in nine patients. **Tables 1** and **2** report the demographic and clinical features of these patients who underwent laparoscopic transperitoneal adrenalectomy.

All patients underwent preoperative biochemical testing and CT and MRI imaging studies. MIBG was used in selected patients. Indications for surgical treatment included: hyperactive adrenal tumors in patients with Conn's syndrome, Cushing's syndrome (**Figure 4**), and pheochromocytoma; and in those patients with non-hyperfunctional adrenal lesions such as cortical adenomas (**Figure 5**), myelolipomas, oncocytomas, and incidentalomas (**Figure 6**).

The operative outcomes for laparasopic adrenalectomy at the authors' institution (**Table 3**) reveal very low conversion, perioperative, and postoperative complication rates. Operative time and blood loss were comparable to results reported in the literature.

Patients	**N = 67**
Functioning neoplasms	35 (52.38%)
Non-functioning neoplasms	32 (47.62%)

Table 1. Functional appearances.

Patients	N = 67	*P value
Age		
Mean (SD)	50.87 (14.40)	0.295
Median	51.25	
Range	20–73	
BMI		
Mean (SD)	26.16 (3.84)	0.393
Median	25.5	
Range	19.5–33	
ASA score		
Mean (SD)	1.50 (0.67)	0.245
Median	1	
Range	I–III	

*P value obtained from Mann-Whitney U test.

Table 2. Demographic and clinical features.

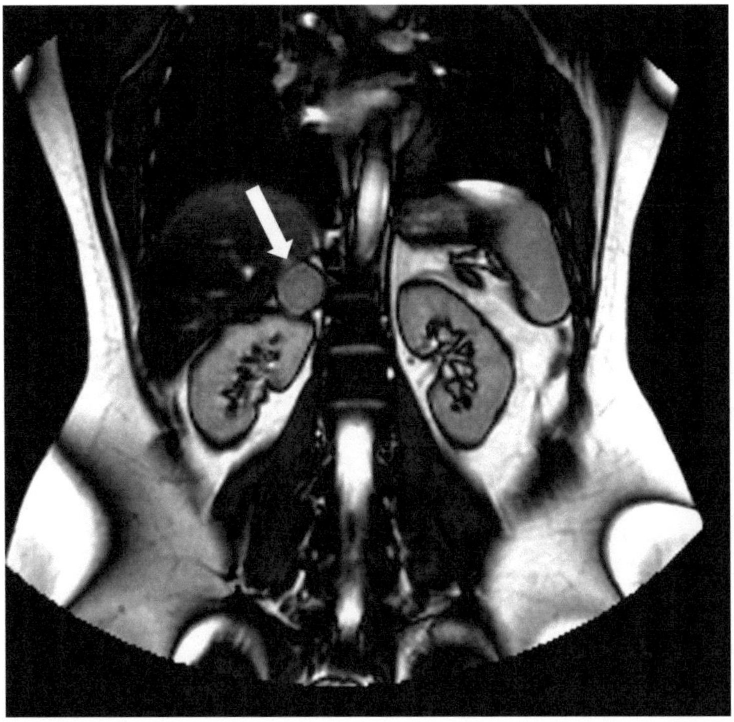

Figure 4. MRI: right adrenal adenoma (Cushing's syndrome).

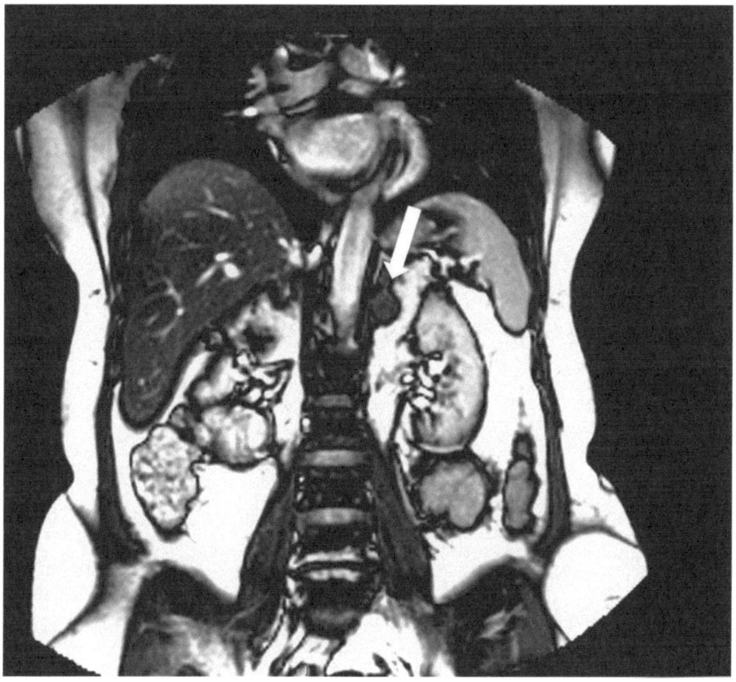

Figure 5. MRI: left adrenal cortical adenoma.

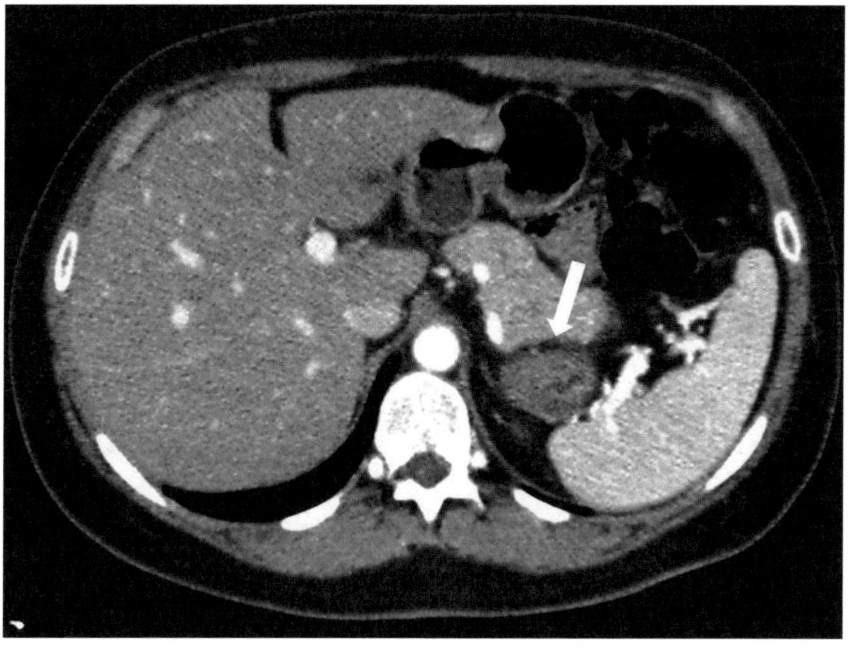

Figure 6. CT: left adrenal incidentaloma.

Patients	N = 67	*P value
Operative time (min)		
Mean (SD)	143 (34.27)	0.012
Median	138.75	
Range	105–210	
Blood loss (ml)		
Mean (SD)	87.22 (33.50)	0.006
Median	82	
Range	50–188	
Conversion rate (%)	5/67 (7%)	0.116
Gland size (cm)		
Mean (SD)	5.81 (1.37)	0.168
Median	5.5	
Range	3.7–9	
Tumor size (cm)		
Mean (SD)	3.13 (1.49)	0.113
Median	2.8	
Range	1.15–6.5	
Postoperative ambulation (hours)		
Mean (SD)	31.25 (8.94)	0.142
Median	27.75	
Range	22–47.5	
Hospital stay (days)		
Mean (SD)	4.05 (1.09)	0.452
Median	4	
Range	3–6	
Perioperative complication rate (%)	1/67 (2%)	0.5
Postoperative complication rate (%)	6/67 (9%)	0.697

*P value obtained from Mann-Whitney U-test (operative time, blood loss, gland size, tumor size, postoperative ambulation, and postoperative hospitalization) and Fisher exact test (conversion, perioperative complication and postoperative complication).

Table 3. Intraoperative and postoperative results of laparoscopic adrenalectomy.

The authors prefer laparoscopic transperitoneal lateral adrenectomy for all patients with adrenal diseases. In their opinion, the laparoscopic transperitoneal and retroperitoneal approaches are essentially equivalent in relation to the surgical skill and surgeon experience.

Choice of the procedure is strongly influenced by the background training of the surgeon. The transperitoneal access allows for complete dissection and control of the adrenal mass and its vascular supply. Most important is the careful dissection of the right adrenal gland that is partially retrocaval with a short adrenal vein that flows directly into the inferior vena cava posterolaterally. Surgical dissection on right side involves close proximity of the liver, duodenum, and right kidney.

Anatomic structures around the left adrenal gland can make dissection difficult. The left adrenal gland is in close proximity with the tail of the pancreas and spleen; the splenopancreatic complex should be widely mobilized and, in some cases, mobilization of the splenic flexure of the colon may be required for adequate exposure of the left adrenal gland. In contrast to the right, along left adrenal vein usually flows into the left renal vein. Some variations of this venous supply can occur (5–6% of cases) and can predispose to intraoperative bleeding [71]. The authors customarily place a drain at the end of their procedure.

For large adrenal tumors, lateral, superior, and inferior dissection of the mass is initially performed because earlier mobilization of the gland can allow easier access to the adrenal vein. More recent surgical devices for dissection and hemostasis have been useful in reducing operative time, but are not essential in the performance of successful adrenalectomy. At their institution, the authors routinely use a monobipolar scalpel and mechanical clips for hemostasis during adrenalectomies that have provided satisfactory results.

6. Conclusion

Minimally invasive adrenalectomy is the preferred surgical treatment of adrenal tumors at many specialized medical centers worldwide. The laparoscopic transabdominal lateral operative technique is most commonly performed. The choice of laparoscopic transabdominal or retroperitoneal adrenalectomy is strongly influenced by background training, skill, and experience of the surgeon. Two issues that constantly evolve with minimally invasive adrenalectomy are a size limit of adrenal mass and appropriateness for malignant adrenal tumors. Some relative limits to laparoscopic adrenalectomy are adrenal tumors >9 cm. Contraindication to minimally invasive adrenalectomy is determined by local neoplastic invasiveness outside the adrenal gland capsule into the periadrenal fat usually delineated by preoperative CT and MRI imaging studies.

Author details

Pasquale Cianci, Alberto Fersini, Nicola Tartaglia, Sabino Capuzzolo, Libero Luca Giambavicchio, Antonio Ambrosi and Vincenzo Neri*

*Address all correspondence to: vincenzo.neri@unifg.it

Department of Medical and Surgical Sciences, University of Foggia, Foggia, Italy

References

[1] Sing PK, Buch HN. Adrenal incidentaloma: Evaluation and management. Journal of Clinical Pathology. 2008;**61**:1168–1173

[2] Bovio S, Cataldi A, Raimondo G, et al. Prevalence of adrenal incidentaloma in a contemporary computerized tomography series. Journal of Endocrinological Investigation. 2006;**29**:298–302

[3] Arnaldi G, Angeli A, Atkinson AB, et al. Diagnosis and complications of Cushing's Syndrome: A consensus statement. The Journal of Clinical Endocrinology & Metabolism. 2003;**88**:5593–5602

[4] Young WF Jr. Minireview: Primary aldosteronism changing concepts in diagnosis and treatment. Endocrinology. 2003;**144**:2208–2213

[5] Bravo EL, Tagle R. Pheochromocytoma: State of the art and future prospects. Endocrine Reviews. 2003;**24**:539–553

[6] Kapoor A, Morris T, Rebello R. Guidelines for the management of the incidentally discovered adrenal mass. Canadian Urological Association Journal. 2011;**5**:241–247

[7] Boland GW, Blake MH, Hahn PF, et al. Incidental adrenal lesions: principles, techniques and algorithms for imaging characterization. Radiology. 2008;**249**:756–775

[8] Hamrahian HH, Ioachimescu AG, Remer EM, et al. Clinical utility of noncontrast computed tomography attenuation value (Hounsfield units) to differentiate adrenal adenomas/hyperplasias from nonadenomas: Cleveland clinic experience. The Journal of Clinical Endocrinology and Metabolism. 2005;**90**: 871–877

[9] Sturgeon C, Shen WT, Clark OH, et al. Risk assessment in 457 adrenal cortical carcinoma; how much does tumor size predict the likelihood of malignancy? Journal of the American College of Surgeons. 2006;**202**:423–430

[10] Thompson L. Pheochromocytoma of the adrenal gland scaled score (PASS) to separate benign from malignant neoplasms. The American Journal of Surgical Pathology. 2002;**26**:551–566

[11] Fernandez MR, Pallares PB, Menendez Torre E, et al. Pheochromocytoma of the adrenal gland scaled score (PASS) as a predictor of aggressive biologic behavior. Endocrine Abstract 2010; 22P44—12th European Congress Endocrinology; 22–28 April 2010; Prague

[12] Machado NO, Qadhi H, Wahaibi K, et al. Laparoscopic adrenalectomy for large adrenocortical carcinoma. Journal of the Society of Laparoendoscopic Surgeons. 2015;**19**(3)-e2015.00036

[13] Porpiglia F, Destefanis P, Fiori C, et al. Does adrenal mass size really affect safety and effectiveness of laparoscopic adrenalectomy? Urology. 2002;**60**:801–805

[14] Kelebew E, Siperstein AE, Clark OH, et al. Results of laparoscopic adrenalectomy for suspected and unsuspected malignant adrenal neoplasms. Archives of Surgery. 2002;**137**: 948–951

[15] Walz MK, Petersenn S, Koch JA, et al. Endoscopic treatment of large primary adrenal tumors. British Journal of Surgery. 2005;**92**:719–723

[16] Palazzo FF, Sebag F, Sierra M, et al. Long-term outcome following laparoscopic adrenalectomy for large solid adrenal cortex tumors. World Journal of Surgery. 2006;**30**:893–898

[17] Ramacciato G, Mercantini P, La Torre M, et al. Is laparoscopic adrenalectomy safe and effective for adrenal masses larger than 7 cm? Surgical Endoscopy. 2008;**22**:516–521

[18] Porpiglia F, Miller BS, Manfredi M, et al. A debate on laparoscopic versus open adrenalectomy for adrenocortical carcinoma. Hormones and Cancer. 2011;**2**(6):372–377

[19] Latronico AC, Chronsos GP. Extensive personal experience: Adrenocortical tumors. The Journal of Clinical Endocrinology and Metabolism. 1997;**82**:1317–1324

[20] Dackiw AP, Lee JE, Gagel RF, et al. Adrenal cortical carcinoma. World Journal of Surgery. 2001;**25**:914–926

[21] Kebelew E, Duh QY. Benign and malignant pheochromocytoma: Diagnosis, treatment and follow-up. Surgical Oncology Clinics of North America. 1998;**7**:765–789

[22] Kim SH, Brennan MF, Russo P, et al. The role of surgery in the treatment of clinically isolated adrenal metastasis. Cancer. 1998;**82**:389–394

[23] Corcione F, Miranda L, Marzano E, et al. Laparoscopic adrenalectomy for malignant neoplasm: our experience in 15 cases. Surgical Endoscopy. 2005;**19**:841–844

[24] Sun C-Y, Ho Y-F, Ding W-H, et al. Laparoscopic adrenalectomy for adrenal tumors. International Journal of Endocrinology. 2014. DOI: 10.1155/2014/241854

[25] Pedziwiatr M, Wierda KM, Natkanier M, et al. Laparoscopic transperitoneal lateral adrenalectomy for malignant and potentially malignant adrenal tumors. BMC Surgery. 2015;**15**:101–107

[26] Sroka G, Slijper N, Shteinberg D, et al. Laparoscopic adrenalectomy for malignant lesions: Safe and effective! SAGES abstract archive. 2012-SS07-S042

[27] Cobb WS, Kercher KW, Sing RF, et al. Laparoscopic adrenalectomy for malignancy. The American Journal of Surgery. 2005;**189**:405–411

[28] Zografos GN, Vasiliadis G, Farfaras AN, et al. Laparoscopic surgery for malignant adrenal tumors. Journal of the Society of Laparoendoscopic Surgeons. 2009;**13**:196–202

[29] Donatini G, Caiazzo R, Do Cao CD, et al. Long-term survival after adrenalectomy for stage I/II adrenocortical carcinoma (ACC): A retrospective comparative cohort study of laparoscopic versus open approach. Annals of Surgical Oncology. 2014;**21**:284–291

[30] Porpiglia F, Fiori C, Daffara F, et al. Retrospective evaluation of the outcome of open versus laparoscopic adrenalectomy for stage I and II adrenocortical cancer. European Urology. 2010;**57**:873–878

[31] Fossa A, Rosok BI, Kazaryan AM, et al. Laparoscopic versus open surgery in stage I–III adrenocortical carcinoma: A retrospective comparison of 32 patients. Acta Oncologica. 2013;**52**:1771–1777

[32] Lombardi CP, Raffaelli M, De Crea C, et al. Open versus endoscopic adrenalectomy in the treatment of localized (stage I/II) adrenocortical carcinoma: Results of a multiinstitu-itional Italian survey. Surgery. 2012;**152**:1158–1164

[33] Foxius A, Ramboux A, Lefebvre Y, et al. Hazards of laparoscopic adrenalectomy for Conn's adenoma when enthusiasm turns to tragedy. Surgical Endoscopy - Springer. 1999;**13**:715–717

[34] Miller BS, Ammori JB, Gauger PG, et al. Laparoscopic resection is inappropriate in patients with known or suspected adrenocortical carcinoma. World Journal of Surgery. 2010;**34**:1380–1385

[35] Leboulleux S, Deandreis D, AlGhuzlan A, et al. Adrenocortical carcinoma: Is the surgical approach a risk factor of peritoneal carcinomatosis? European Journal of Endocrinology. 2010;**162**:1147–1153

[36] Gagner M, Lacroix A, Bolté E. Laparoscopic adrenalectomy in Cushing's syndrome and pheochromocytoma. The New England Journal of Medicine. 1 Oct 1992;**327**(14):1033

[37] Fernández-Cruz L, Saenz A, Benarroch G, et al. Laparoscopic unilateral and bilateral adrenalectomy for Cushing's syndrome. Transperitoneal and retroperitoneal approaches. Annals of Surgery. 1996;**224**:727–736

[38] Lee J, El-Tamer M, Schifftneretal JB, Inabnet WB, 3rd. Open and laparoscopic adrenalectomy: Analysis of the national surgical quality improvement program. Journal of the American College of Surgeons. 2008;**206**: 953–961

[39] Assalia A, Gagner M. Laparoscopic adrenalectomy. British Journal of Surgery. Oct 2004;**91**(10):1259–1274

[40] Cianci P, Fersini A, Tartaglia N, et al. Are there differences between the right and left laparoscopic adrenalectomy? Our experience. AnnaliItaliani di Chirurgia. 2016;**87**:242–246

[41] Fernández-Cruz L, Saenz A, Taura P, et al. Retroperitoneal approach in laparoscopic adrenalectomy: Is it advantageous? Surgical Endoscopy. Jan 1999;**13**(1):86–90

[42] Takeda M. Laparoscopic adrenalectomy: Transperitoneal vs retroperitoneal approaches. Biomedicine & Pharmacotherapy. 2000;**54**(Suppl 1):207s-210s

[43] Lezoche E, Guerrieri M, Paganini AM, et al. Laparoscopic adrenalectomy by the anterior transperitoneal approach. Results of 108 operations in unselected cases. Surgical Endoscopy. 2000;**14**:920–925

[44] Chiu AW. Laparoscopic retroperitoneal adrenalectomy: Clinical experience with 120 consecutive cases. Asian Journal of Surgery. 2003;**26**:139–144

[45] Bonjer HJ, Sorm V, Berends FJ, et al. Endoscopic retroperitoneal adrenalectomy: Lessons learned from 111 consecutive cases. Annals of Surgery. 2000;**232**:796–803

[46] Gasman D, Droupy S, Koutani A, et al. Laparoscopic adrenalectomy: The retroperitoneal approach. The Journal of Urology. 1998;**156**:1816–1820

[47] Soulié M, Mouly P, Caron P, et al. Retroperitoneal laparoscopic adrenalectomy: Clinical experience in 52 procedures. Urology. 2000;**56**:921–925

[48] Salomon L, Soulié M, Mouly P, et al. Experience with retroperitoneal laparoscopic adrenalectomy in 115 procedures. The Journal of Urology. 2001;**166**:38–41

[49] Fazeli-Matin S, Gill IS, Hsu TH, et al. Laparoscopic renal and adrenal surgery in obese patients: Comparison to open surgery. The Journal of Urology. 1999;**162**:665–670

[50] Wolf JS Jr, Monk TG, McDougall EM, et al. The extraperitoneal approach and subcutaneous emphysema are associated with greater absorption of carbon dioxide during laparoscopic renal surgery. The Journal of Urology. 1995;**154**:959–963

[51] Ng CS, Gill IS, Sung GT, et al. Retroperitoneoscopic surgery was not associated with increased carbon dioxide absorption. The Journal of Urology. 1999;**162**:1268–1271

[52] Walz MK, Alesina PF, Wenger FA, et al. Posterior retroperitoneoscopic adrenalectomy—Results of 560 procedures in 520 patients. Surgery. Dec 2006;**140**(6):943-948;discussion 948-950

[53] Suzuki K, Ihara H, Mugiya S, et al. Complications of laparoscopic adrenalectomy in 75 patients treated by the same surgeon. European Urology. 1999;**36**:40–47

[54] Bennet IC, Ray M. Hand-assisted laparoscopic adrenalectomy: An alternative minimal invasive surgical technique for the adrenal gland. ANZ Journal of Surgery. 2002;**72**:801–805

[55] Mack MJ, Aronoff RJ, Acuff TE, et al. Thoracoscopic transdiaphragmatic approach for adrenal biopsy. The Annals of Thoracic Surgery. 1993;**55**:772–773

[56] Pompeo E, Coosemans W, De Leyn P, et al. Thoracoscopic transdiaphragmatic left adrenalectomy. An experimental study. Surgical Endoscopy. 1997;**11**:390–392

[57] Gill IS, Meraney AM, Thomas JC, et al. Thoracoscopic transdiaphragmatic adrenalectomy: The initial experience. The Journal of Urology. 2001;**165**:1875–1881

[58] Marescaux J, Dallemagne B, Perretta S, et al. Surgery without scars: Report of transluminal cholecystectomy in a human being. Archives of Surgery. Sep 2007;**142**(9):823–826

[59] Perretta S, Allemann P, Asakuma M, et al. Adrenalectomy using natural orifice translumenal endoscopic surgery (NOTES): A transvaginal retroperitoneal approach. Surgical Endoscopy. Jun 2009;**23**(6):1390. DOI: 10.1007/s00464-009-0367-9. Epub 5 Mar 2009

[60] Zou X, Zhang G, Xiao R, et al. Transvaginal natural orifice transluminal endoscopic surgery (NOTES)-assisted laparoscopic adrenalectomy: First clinical experience. Surgical Endoscopy. Dec 2011;**25**(12):3767–3772. DOI: 10.1007/s00464-011-1786-y. Epub.3 Jun 2011

[61] Horgan S, Vanuno D. Robots in laparoscopic surgery. Journal of Laparoendoscopic & Advanced Surgical Techniques. Part A. 2001 Dec;**11**(6):415–419

[62] Young JA, Chapman WH 3rd, Kim VB, Albrecht RJ, Ng PC, Nifong LW, Chitwood WR Jr. Robotic-assisted adrenalectomy for adrenal incidentaloma: Case and review of the technique. Surgical Laparoscopy, Endoscopy & Percutaneous Techniques. Apr 2002;**12**(2):126–130

[63] Hyams ES, Stifelman MD. The role of robotics for adrenal pathology. Current Opinion in Urology. 2009;**19**(1):89–96

[64] Desai MM, Gill IS, Kaouk JH, et al. Robotic-assisted laparoscopic adrenalectomy. Urology. 2002 Dec;**60**(6):1104–1107

[65] Berber E, Mitchell J, Milas M, et al. Robotic posterior retroperitoneal adrenalectomy: operative technique. Archives of Surgery. 2010 Aug;**145**(8):781–784

[66] Merseburger AS, Herrmann TR, Shariat SF, et al. European Association of Urology. EAU guidelines on robotic and single-site surgery in urology. European Urology 2013;**64**:277–291

[67] Brunaud L, Bresler L, Ayav A, et al. Robotic-assisted adrenalectomy: What advantages compared to lateral transperitoneal laparoscopic adrenalectomy? The American Journal of Surgery. 2008;**195**:433–438

[68] Winter JM, Talamini MA, Stanfield CL, et al. Thirty robotic adrenalectomies: A single institution's experience. Surgical Endoscopy. 2006;**20**:119–124

[69] Taskin HE, Berber E. Robotic adrenalectomy. The Cancer Journal. 2013;**19**(2):162–166

[70] Brandao LF, Autorino R, Laydner H, et al. Robotic versus laparoscopic adrenalectomy: A systematic review and meta-analysis. European Urology. 2014;**65**(6):1154–1161

[71] Sebe P, Peyromaure M, Raynand A, et al. Anatomical variations in the drainage of the principal adrenal veins: The results of 88 venograms. Surgical and Radiologic Anatomy. 2002;**24**:222–225

Chapter 8

Sudden Death due to Diseases of the Adrenal Glands and Paraganglia

Silvia Damiana Visonà, Luca Tajana and
Antonio Osculati

Additional information is available at the end of the chapter

http://dx.doi.org/10.5772/intechopen.69416

Abstract

Coroners and pathologists commonly evaluate unexpected deaths due to diseases of the adrenal glands and paraganglia, which are, unfortunately, not rare in their totality. Although cardiac causes are the main cause of sudden death, endocrine conditions can produce sudden, unexpected deaths that need further investigation, especially in younger patients. This chapter focuses on the issue of sudden death due to diseases involving adrenal glands and paraganglia. The main causes of sudden death due to adrenal gland pathology will be examined, paying particular attention to the pathophysiology of sudden death, macroscopic and microscopic characteristics and their correlation with clinical features. These issues are of great interest, especially considering the clinical impact of sudden death and its rarity among patients with adrenal gland diseases. The forensic pathologist's examination is extremely important in determining the cause of death and findings not clinically observable and can contribute to the improvement of the clinical and surgical approach in treating such patients.

Keywords: adrenal glands, paraganglia, sudden death, Addison's disease, Cushing's syndrome, pheochromocytoma, paraganglioma

1. Introduction

Coroners and pathologists are frequently presented with unexpected and sudden deaths, which are, unfortunately, not rare. The definition of sudden death suggested by the World Health Organization is a death occurring within 24 h from the onset of symptoms. However, for most clinicians and pathologists, this interval is too long with many regarding sudden death within one hour from the onset of illness [1]. Cardiovascular, central nervous system and respiratory diseases account for the majority of unexpected natural deaths. Heart diseases are the main cause of sudden death and most investigated. However, in cases of an unexpected death in young and apparently healthy patients, many other medical conditions need to be considered.

Forensic pathologists have a pivotal role in investigating sudden deaths, as autopsies are often performed. One reason is that in many jurisdictions, death may only be certified by an attending physician if he or she has recently seen the patient and it is clear that their death was caused by a potentially lethal disease. When death cannot be certified by an attending physician, the patient case is referred for medicolegal investigation. Under these circumstances, the role of the forensic pathologist is twofold: to determine the cause and manner of death and initiate a multidisciplinary process in order to prevent further deaths in existing family members (especially in the case of familial diseases) or in other patients suffering from a similar disorder. Lastly, an autopsy is often ordered by a prosecutor if medical malpractice is suspected, especially if the death occurred at a hospital.

The forensic pathologist's examination is extremely important since providing a cause of death and other findings previously not known can contribute to the improvement of clinical and surgical management of such patients, and help avoid this undesired outcome in other similar cases. Sudden deaths from adrenal diseases are rare compared to other causes, extremely difficult to recognize clinically, and often discovered at autopsy by thorough postmortem investigations.

In this chapter, diseases of the adrenal gland and paraganglia that can cause sudden death will be discussed, including the clinical correlation and pattern, as well as the mechanism and presentation of death.

2. Corticoadrenal hypofunction and sudden death

When dealing with a sudden death in an otherwise healthy individual, adrenocortical insufficiency should always be considered. This condition is very difficult to recognize clinically, since signs and symptoms are nonspecific, and as such, it is often encountered in forensic practice, as the cause of unexpected death. A careful investigation of the adrenal glands is essential, especially if underlying diseases of the cardiovascular and nervous system exists. An autopsy is commonly ordered when medical mistakes are suspected including late or misdiagnosis. In such circumstances, assessment of clinical condition before death, when possible, through an accurate anamnesis collected from the relatives of the decedent, and their correlation with the macroscopic and microscopic postmortem pattern is paramount.

Adrenal insufficiency is an infrequent cause of sudden death and occurs most frequently in individuals treated for other critical conditions where impairment of corticoadrenal function often occurs. Nevertheless, it is well known that adrenal insufficiency can remain clinically silent until abrupt adrenal decompensation takes place and the patient dies suddenly. In fact, >90% of the adrenal cortex bilaterally must be nonfunctional before any clinical manifestation by infective, inflammatory, or neoplastic processes manifests and causes sudden death [2].

http://dx.doi.org/10.5772/intechopen.69416

Both Addison's disease (primary corticoadrenal insufficiency due to bilateral destruction or damage to the adrenal cortex) and secondary hypocortisolism (ACTH hypoproduction) result in the lack of hormone production that can lead to sudden death. Regardless of the cause, the acute adrenal crisis is characterized by a shock-like condition due to electrolyte deficit with acidosis, vomiting, diarrhea, hemorrhage, and numbness. Death is often caused by hyponatremia, the result of aldosterone deficiency, leading to cerebral and pulmonary edema.

Forensic pathologists may encounter cases of decedents with already known Addison's disease in which an unknown stress, such as superimposed disease or a stimulating event, has triggered a lethal adrenal crisis. In such instances, it can be challenging to identify the precipitating event, which most commonly is an infection or surgical procedure [2].

At autopsy, decedents who suffered from chronic adrenocortical insufficiency are often slim and cachectic with a brownish skin pigmentation also seen in anorexia nervosa. Generally, pathologic findings at autopsy may include a low combined weight and atrophy making the adrenal glands difficult to detect. For this reason, multiple slides of the fatty tissue surrounding the superior pole of each kidney should be taken for histologic examination. The microscopic appearance of adrenal gland tissue shows atrophy of adrenal cortical cells, and a collapsed vascular reticulin framework (**Figures 1** and **2**).

Only a few sudden deaths due to an endocrine imbalance in an individual previously known to have been treated for adrenocortical insufficiency are found in the literature. A reported case of a 50-year-old man, whose medical history was significant for Addison's disease, was found dead in a hotel room [3]. Taking into account this man's circumstances, medical history, and

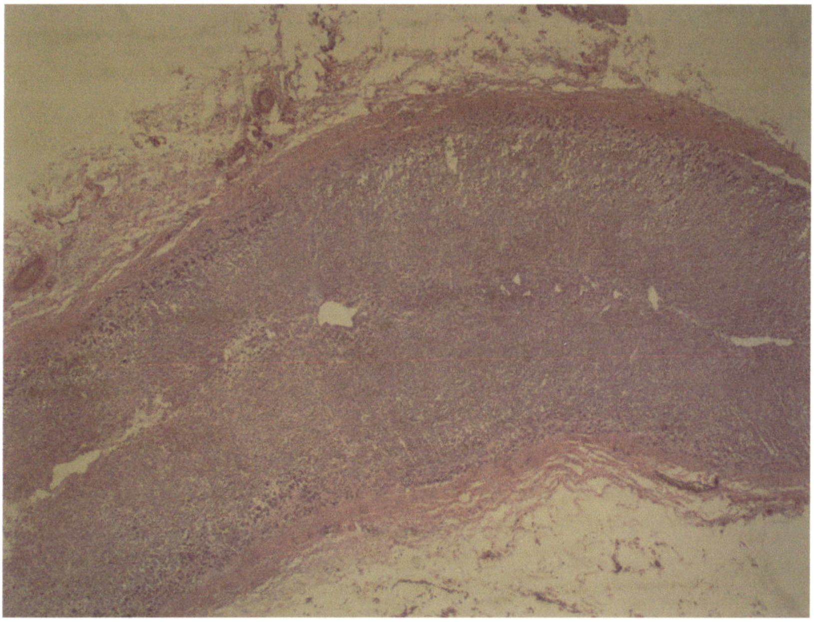

Figure 1. Atrophy of the adrenal cortex (secondary to cranioencephalic trauma), H&E, 12×.

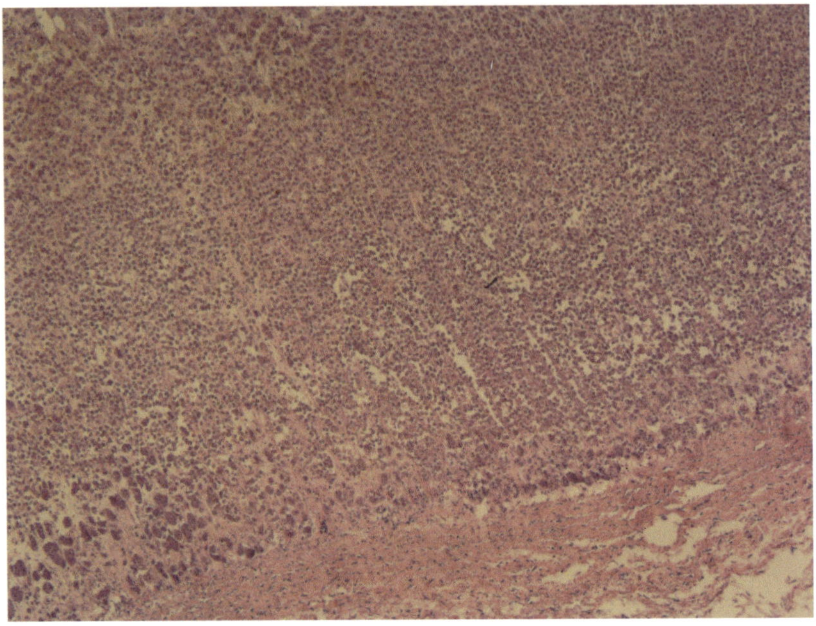

Figure 2. Atrophy of the adrenal cortex (secondary to cranioencephalic trauma) H&E, 60×.

autopsy findings, cause of death was attributed to acute adrenal crisis secondary to gland hypofunction and insufficiency. Adrenocortical insufficiency can be due to many causes including autoimmune gland destruction, infection, and hemorrhage.

2.1. Autoimmune adrenalitis

In industrialized countries, adrenal insufficiency is mostly caused by an autoimmune disease that is particularly challenging to evaluate in postmortem investigation as typical macroscopic findings reveal difficult to detect adrenal glands with markedly reduced size [2]. Histologically, in autoimmune adrenalitis, adrenal glands show significant reduction of cortical parenchyma and lymphocytic and plasma cell infiltration (almost exclusively in the cortical region) associated with the destruction of cortical cells. The major difference between Addison's disease caused by tuberculosis and autoimmune adrenalitis is that in the former, there is the destruction of the whole gland, whereas in the latter, only the cortex is involved. Typically, the dimension of the adrenal glands is markedly reduced and sometimes undetectable. Microscopically, the cortex is generally atrophied and replaced by islands of large eosinophilic cells, but no fibrosis is seen, even though the residual vascular reticulin framework can be observed. Occasionally, there is moderate infiltration, mainly composed by lymphocytes, with some involvement of the medulla that is otherwise normal. Inflammation is often accompanied by fibrosis [4]. Histologic features seen in autoimmune adrenalitis include the enlargement of surviving cells that also show nuclear atypia, probably due to prolonged ACTH stimulation [2].

There are a few cases describing autoimmune adrenalitis as a cause of sudden death in the literature. In one case report, a 12-year-old girl hospitalized following a 2-day history of recurrent vomiting was given the misdiagnosis of diabetic ketoacidosis [5]. She died shortly after hospitalization. The diagnosis of autoimmune Addison's disease was rendered at autopsy based on histology. Microscopic examination revealed depletion and atrophy of the adrenal cortex with enlargement, eosinophilia of surviving cortical cells, and prominent round cell infiltrates composed mostly of lymphocytes. In addition, there was mild chronic lymphocytic thyroiditis. Other organs were unremarkable except for marked pulmonary congestion and edema with early basal pneumonic changes and cerebral edema.

Undeniably, histopathology is essential for the diagnosis of autoimmune adrenalitis, and examination of postmortem blood, particularly of serum cortisol levels, should be included in the investigation. The availability of appropriately stored antemortem serum samples is of great importance, and cortisol is sufficiently stable in postmortem blood [6]. Levels of cortisol, 17-hydroxycorticosterone, aldosterone, and dehydroepiandrosterone in postmortem serum from femoral blood and urine (in combination with other biochemical investigation) allow for the differentiation between ketoacidosis and adrenocortical insufficiency [7]. An additional examination for adrenal autoantibodies on postmortem serum can be conducted [2].

2.2. Tuberculosis and other infections involving adrenal glands

About 10% of Addison's disease cases have an infectious etiology [8]. HIV/AIDS and opportunistic infections such as cytomegalovirus are the most commonly cited causes, following tuberculosis. Currently, adrenal tuberculosis has generally considered a disease of immigrants from endemic areas, immunocompromised or destitute individuals. In the past, tuberculosis was the most common cause of adrenocortical insufficiency and remains the primary cause in the developing countries where it accounts for about 20–30% of cases of Addison's disease. Various fungi including *Cryptococcus, Histoplasma, Coccidioides*, and *Paracoccidioides* also infect the adrenal glands as reported in several published case reports. It is well known that *Mycobacterium tuberculosis* complex spreads to the adrenal glands hematogenously. Clinical manifestations may take 3 years to become apparent, and asymptomatic infection is not uncommon [8].

The only case report, to the authors' knowledge, of sudden death due to isolated adrenal tuberculosis was reported in 1985 [9]. The patient with a history of a disseminated carcinoma of the prostate presented with normal blood pressure, lack of skin pigmentation, and normal electrolytes. He died suddenly after being admitted to a hospital for investigation of pleural thickening. The autopsy revealed that his adrenal glands were both completely replaced by caseous material containing acid-fast bacilli. There was no evidence of tuberculosis in any other organs.

Another important issue regarding the adrenal glands concerns HIV infection. Apart from direct infection, opportunistic infections and antiretroviral medications also have a significant effect on the adrenal glands. Adrenal insufficiency is prevalent in 17% of patients admitted with AIDS [10]. In a forensic context, when dealing with an unexpected death in a subject previously known as having HIV, adrenal insufficiency should be considered and properly investigated.

The histopathology and morphologic assessment of the adrenal glands were investigated in 128 autopsied patients who died from AIDS [11]. Interestingly, alteration of the adrenal glands was observed in 99.2% of these decedents with various patterns of disease and different pathogens. Inflammatory infiltrates, mostly with a predominance of mononuclear cells, were observed in 99.2% of the cases. The medulla was almost always involved. Fibrosis, necrosis, neoplasia, and hemorrhage were also detected.

Human cytomegalovirus (CMV) has been frequently identified as a cause of adrenal insufficiency, especially in patients with HIV/AIDS. In one report, CMV-infected normal human adrenocortical cells and induced cytopathic changes [12]. CMV also acts as an inducer of steroidogenesis, which may explain the discordance between the high rates of CMV adrenalitis in immunosuppressed patients in autopsy studies and the relatively rare diagnosis of adrenal insufficiency antemortem. Interestingly, while adrenalitis may be the sole manifestation, the disease is usually disseminated. CMV typically affects the cortex-medulla junction [11].

Many other rare infections can affect the adrenal glands. Addisonian crisis has been reported in patients afflicted with such pathogens as: *histoplasma capsulatum* (commonly in HIV patients with clinical manifestation similar to tuberculosis), *paracoccidiomycosis* (endemic in several South American countries where adrenal insufficiency has been reported in 2.9–48.2% of patients), viruses (herpes simplex, Epstein Barr, CMV), and, very rarely, other bacteria and parasites [8].

2.3. Hemorrhage

Among the causes of adrenal insufficiency, bilateral adrenal hemorrhage is most frequently encountered in forensic practice. It is of particular interest because it is often clinically silent until the patient's condition worsens abruptly and results in sudden death. Various clinical signs and symptoms occur in the early stages of adrenal hemorrhage, including sudden or gradual back pain, epigastralgia and nonspecific conditions such as fatigue, fever, tachycardia, nausea, vomiting, dizziness, and hypotension. Adrenal insufficiency may also exhibit hyponatraemia, hyperkalemia, and hypoglycemia due to increased ACTH and decreased cortisol levels.

Bilateral adrenal hemorrhage can be due to many causes and can be classified as traumatic or nontraumatic. The exact mechanism of nontraumatic adrenal hemorrhage is still unclear. Adrenal vascularities are referred to as an 'adrenal dam' because adrenal glands have sufficient vascularity, but easily become hemorrhagic and embolic due to their anatomical configuration. An extremely high rate of blood flow, the arterial network that abruptly transitions to a capillary plexus, and, above all, the drainage by a single, central vein are certainly anatomical factors of importance [13].

Most cases of nontraumatic adrenal hemorrhage are related to stress due to infection, sepsis (Waterhouse-Friderichsen syndrome), surgery, thermal injuries, coagulopathic and thromboembolic disorders, neonatal stress, tumor metastasis to the adrenal glands [14], antiphospholipid syndrome [15], or idiopathic [16]. Interestingly, adrenal hemorrhage resulting in acute adrenal insufficiency has been reported to be a rare complication of anticoagulant therapy [17].

Bilateral adrenal hemorrhage has also been reported as a life-threatening complication of anaphylactic shock [18].

Adrenal hemorrhage at autopsy is not necessarily associated with sepsis, although it is the most frequent cause. This pathologic finding is much more common as a contributor to mortality, and a significant number of ill patients could be saved if such diagnosis was suspected antemortem. As they reside in a relatively protected location of the retroperitoneum, adrenal gland hemorrhage related to trauma is usually associated with other conspicuous intra-abdominal injuries [13].

In septic patients, the involvement of the adrenal glands seems to have a critical role in determining prognosis. A Mayo Clinic study revealed that corticosteroid treatment in situations of severe stress or sepsis had little effect on outcome (9% vs. 6% survival with and without corticosteroid treatment, respectively), in sharp contrast to adrenal hemorrhage occurring postoperatively as well as in the antiphospholipid-antibody syndrome [19]. In a study conducted on mice, there was a strong and significant correlation between mortality and adrenal inflammation, but not with plasma cytokine concentration or systemic inflammation [20]. This study demonstrated that adrenal inflammation during sepsis is associated with increased cell death, adrenal hemorrhage, and inadequate ACTH response.

The majority of reports cite massive adrenal hemorrhage as the most common nontraumatic cause of sudden death associated with sepsis, which is consistent with the authors' experience. Adrenal hemorrhage and insufficiency is classically associated with meningococcemia as part of the Waterhouse-Friderichsen syndrome. This catastrophic syndrome is characterized by overwhelming bacterial infection, classically *Neisseria meningitidis* septicemia, but also caused by other highly virulent organisms, e.g. *Haemophilus influenzae*, hemolytic *streptococcus*, and *pneumococcus* [21]. Patients typically present with a sudden onset of a rapidly progressive illness and hypotension leading to shock, cyanosis, petechial rash, rapidly developing adrenocortical insufficiency associated with massive bilateral adrenal hemorrhage, and death usually within 24 h [13, 21]. In spite of treatment with sulphonamides, antibiotics, and steroids, the prognosis is still extremely poor.

Examining the autopsy records from their institution, the authors found six patient cases in which adrenal hemorrhage was the cause of a sudden death. The age incidence varied from a 40-week old fetus to a 45-year-old man described as follows:

(1) A 1-year-old child with a few hour history of high fever referred to a hospital for difficulty breathing; he arrived dead at the hospital. Histology showed bilateral, massive adrenal hemorrhages. *Meningococci* were isolated from blood cultures performed before death.

(2) A 45-year-old man, with a 12-hour history of diarrhea and vomiting, suddenly died at the Emergency Department that he visited for a purple spot on his forehead. Postmortem examination revealed massive bilateral adrenal hemorrhage, but no microorganism was isolated.

(3) A 19-year-old man, with high fever of a few hours, arrived dead at the hospital. No microorganisms were isolated, but the postmortem histopathology revealed massively hemorrhagic adrenal glands, cerebral and meningeal hyperemia, and spots.

(4) Intrauterine fetal death of a fetus at term (40 weeks of gestation) due to *Streptococcus agalactiae* sepsis. Histopathology showed complete hemorrhagic necrosis of both adrenal glands.

(5) A 6-month-old girl who was brought to the Emergency Department with a high fever, and after few hours later, suddenly died.

(6) A 28-year-old woman who died suddenly from fulminant meningitis.

This case of the 28-year-old woman who died from fulminant meningitis is of particular interest because of the typical fulminant presentation. Her anamnesis was completely negative. She was admitted to the Emergency Department presenting with fever, rigors, nausea, and vomiting. A physical examination performed revealed no significant findings, except for abdominal tenderness and inflammation of the pharynx. The patient was discharged, but she persisted in having a high fever (40°C) and vomiting. She returned to the same hospital and was admitted to the Department of Medicine. At the time of admission, blood samples were taken for microbiological testing, and antibiotic therapy (3 g of ampicillin and 2 g of cefotaxime) was administered. About 2 h after admission, the woman became hypotensive, had difficulty breathing, and developed mild rigor nuchalis and diffuse petechiae. She was brought to the Intensive Care Unit, where she died 2 h later. Group C *N. meningitidis* was detected in her blood cultures taken before death. At autopsy, massive bilateral adrenal hemorrhage and diffuse petechiae were identified. Bacterial cultures of the postmortem blood samples (confirmed by PCR analysis) confirmed the woman's death due to fulminant sepsis from group C *N. meningitidis*.

Another characteristic case involves a 6-month-old girl who presented to the Emergency Department with a high fever (up to 39°C). A few hours later, she developed cyanosis and dyspnea and died suddenly. At forensic autopsy, performed 7 days after death, macroscopic examination revealed pulmonary edema and bilateral adrenal hemorrhage (**Figures 3–5**).

Before an autopsy, blood (from neck vessels) and cerebrospinal fluid (through lumbar puncture) samples were collected with a sterile technique for subsequent microbiologic examination. *N. meningitidis* grew in cultures of blood and cerebrospinal fluid samples after incubation for 48 h, thus providing the postmortem diagnosis of sepsis due to *N. meningitidis*. The main microscopic finding was massive hemorrhage of the adrenal glands (**Figures 6** and **7**).

Premortem diagnosis was not possible because the fulminant disease had caused the baby to die too quickly. Indeed, detection of *N. meningitidis* in postmortem cultures determined the cause of death.

The two aforementioned case reports are worthy of attention because they demonstrate the rapid course of Waterhouse-Friderichsen syndrome, leading to sudden death before a clinical or microbiologic diagnosis can be made. Diagnosis of adrenal hemorrhage is often complicated by its nonspecific presentation, but it should nevertheless be considered as a possible cause of back pain in the setting of an acute illness, especially in the absence of other obvious causes. Appropriate hydrocortisone replacement therapy should be based on the patient's symptoms and their daily needs. Moreover, individuals with adrenal insufficiency should be made aware of how to detect an imminent adrenal crisis, and how to adjust their dose of hydrocortisone accordingly [17]. Although prognosis can be extremely poor, if a proper diagnosis is promptly rendered, the patient can be successfully treated [16].

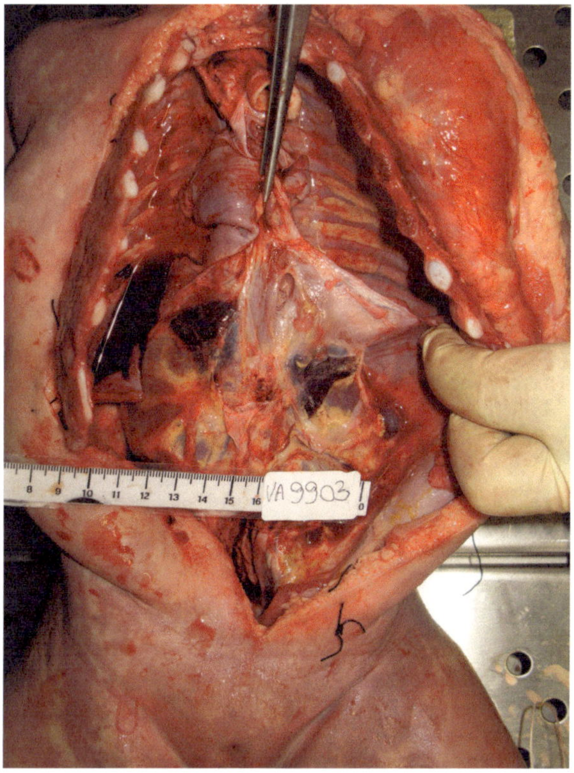

Figure 3. Hemorrhagic adrenal glands before their isolation and removal.

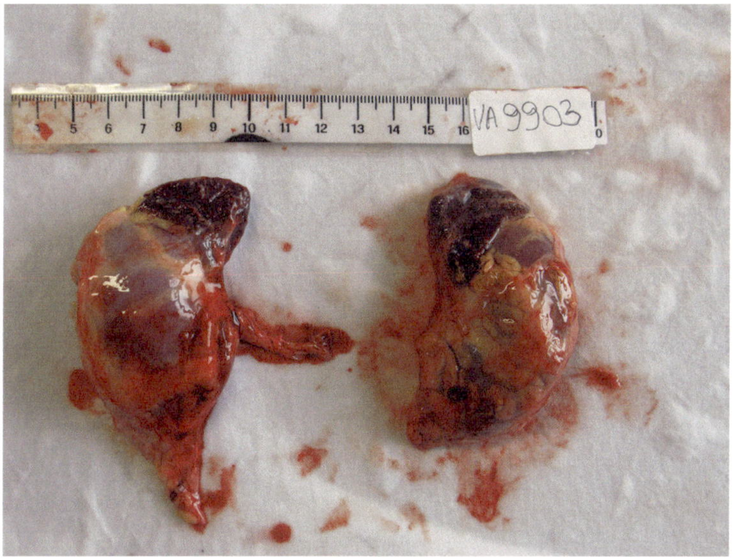

Figure 4. Hemorrhagic adrenal glands before their isolation from the kidneys.

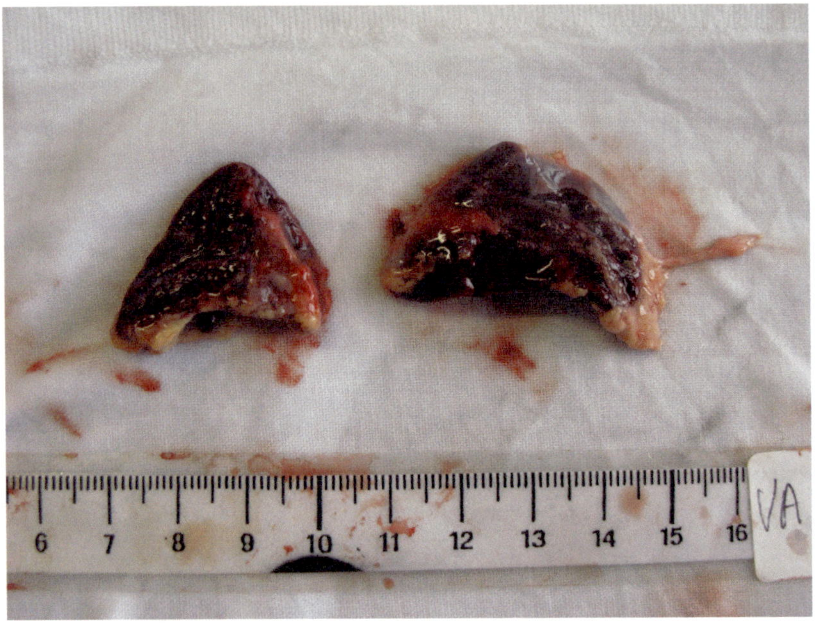

Figure 5. Isolated hemorrhagic adrenal glands.

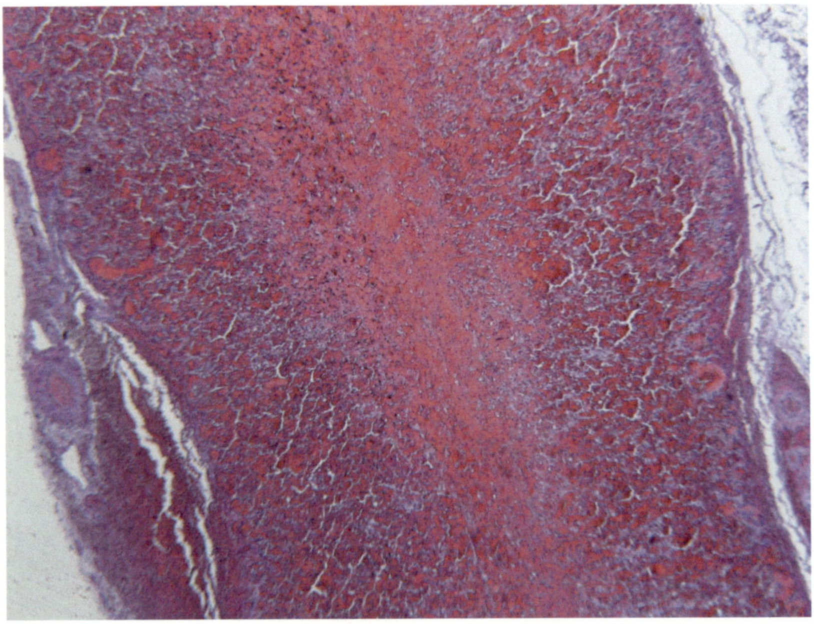

Figure 6. Massive hemorrhage of the adrenal glands, H&E, 12×.

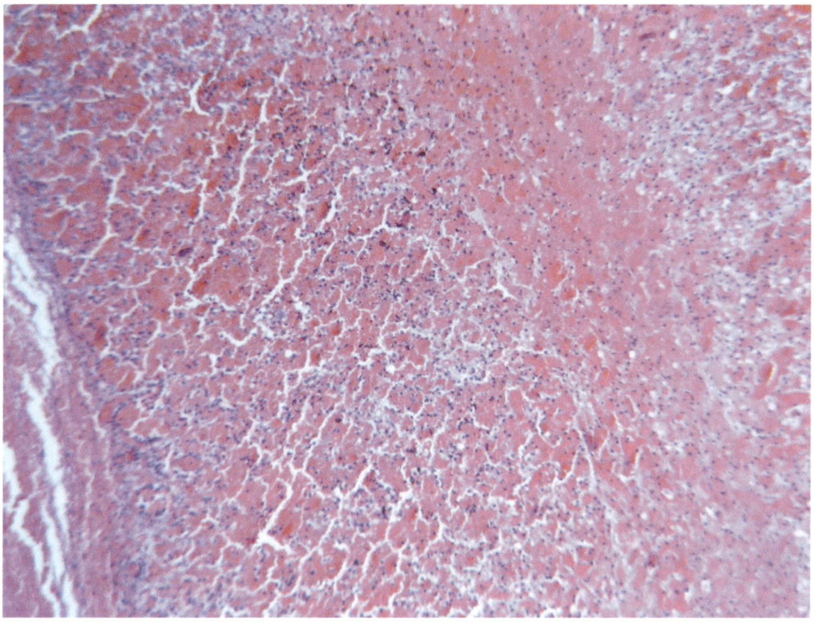

Figure 7. Massive hemorrhage of the adrenal glands, H&E, 60×.

3. Hypercortisolism

Cushing's disease and syndrome are associated with an increased morbidity compared to the general population, related to central obesity, insulin resistance, diabetes mellitus, hypertension, hyperlipidemia and osteoporosis, all due to cortisol hypersecretion. There is also an increased cardiovascular risk profile. Moreover, psychiatric disorders have been documented in these patients, ranging from anxiety to major depression [22]. The immunosuppressive effect of cortisol is also associated with an increased susceptibility to infections. Regarding children, despite advances in early diagnosis and treatment of pediatric Cushing's syndrome, a 2.5% mortality rate was identified in a recent study carried out in a large cohort of children referred to an experienced, tertiary care referral center for this condition [23].

Sudden death due to Cushing's disease is very rare but occasionally reported in the literature. In one case report, a woman with previously suspected Cushing's disease presented with atypical psychosis followed by sudden death [24]. The death occurred while the patient was undergoing clinical studies in an endocrine unit, because of suspected Cushing's disease based on physical examination revealing abdominal striae, hirsutism, amenorrhea, acne and buffalo hump, biochemical studies demonstrating hypercortisolism, and CT scan revealing enlarged adrenal glands. An autopsy revealed a small chronic ulcer in the gastric antrum with acute extension into an artery. A basophil pituitary adenoma was also noted weighing 2.1 g. The adrenal glands were both hyperplasic weighing 10 g. The cause of death was determined to be gastrointestinal bleed from an acute ulcer, which was related to the Cushing's disease.

In another interesting case report, a patient was resuscitated from three episodes of ventricular fibrillation secondary to serious hypokalemia caused by lung carcinoma secreting adrenocorticotropic hormone (ACTH) [25]. This description represents another potential cause of sudden death in patients who may have Cushing's syndrome, which may cause multiple clinical and biochemical derangements.

These two case reports highlight sudden death among patients with differing presentations of Cushing's disease and syndrome. Postmortem investigations are of great importance in determining the cause of death, in which Cushing's syndrome might be previously unknown, and its presentation atypical. Among the causes of sudden death, hypercortisolism must be excluded. It is essential to note the clinical presentation of Cushing's, which includes moon facies, buffalo hump, purple abdominal striae, truncal obesity, hirsutism, weight gain, hypertension, diabetes, and muscular weakness. Typical autopsy findings include enlargement of the pituitary gland and/or the adrenal glands. Alterations encountered in the adrenal glands, in order of frequency, reveal diffuse or isolated hyperplasia (always bilateral), adenoma or carcinoma (usually unilateral). Microscopic examinations are also essential to render the postmortem diagnosis [38].

4. Tumors

Among those that affect the adrenal glands, neuroendocrine tumors are strongly related to the sudden death of patients, characterized by adrenaline or noradrenaline secretion with dire consequences on the cardiovascular system. Other neoplasms can cause Addison's disease in patients, potentially leading to sudden death, because they replace the entire parenchyma of the adrenal gland. Adrenal involvement by tumors arising from other sites most commonly causes adrenal insufficiency.

An interesting example of a benign adrenal tumor that can lead to sudden death is a myelolipoma (**Figures 8–10**).

Myelolipoma is a tumor-like growth composed of mature fat tissue and bone marrow elements that occur in adrenal glands as an isolated soft tissue mass. These benign tumors may be associated with endocrine disorders such as hermaphroditism, Cushing's disease, Addison's disease, and obesity of unknown cause. Although giant myelolipomas have been reported in the literature, these tumors rarely measure >5 cm [26].

4.1. Pheochromocytomas and paragangliomas

Pheochromocytomas and paragangliomas are neuroendocrine tumors derived from chromaffin cells. Generally, they are rare with a prevalence estimated between 1:6500 and 1:2500, and an annual incidence in the United States of 500–1600 cases per year [27]. In patients with hypertension, they occur in about 0.05–0.1% of them. However, half of all patients have paroxysmal hypertension or normotension, and this probably accounts for only 50% of people harboring pheochromocytoma or paraganglioma. Moreover, their incidence may be even

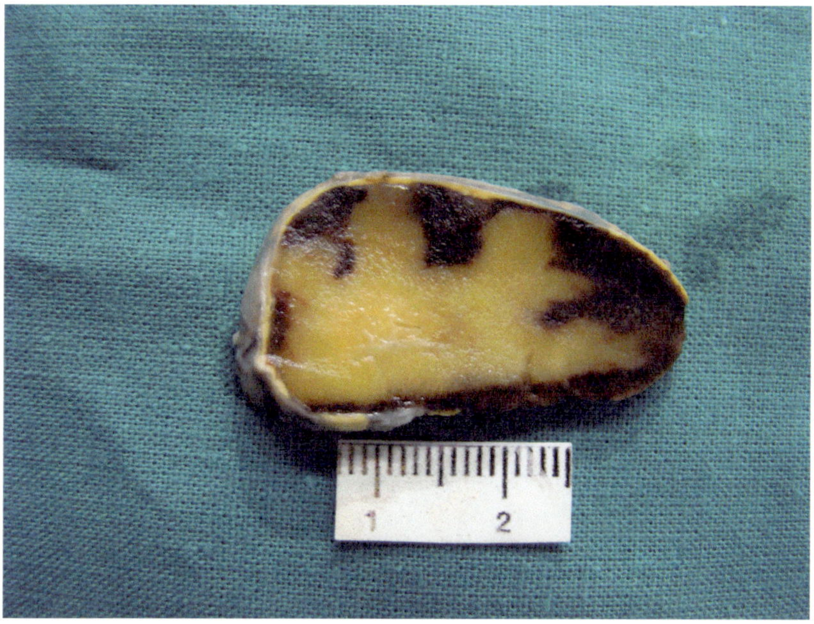

Figure 8. Macroscopic appearance of myelolipoma.

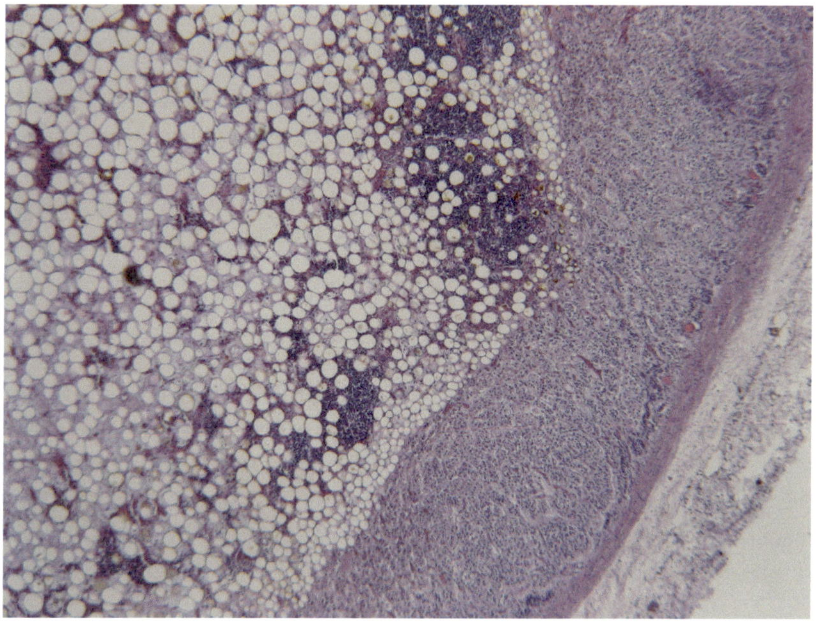

Figure 9. Microscopic appearance of myelolipoma, H&E, 60×.

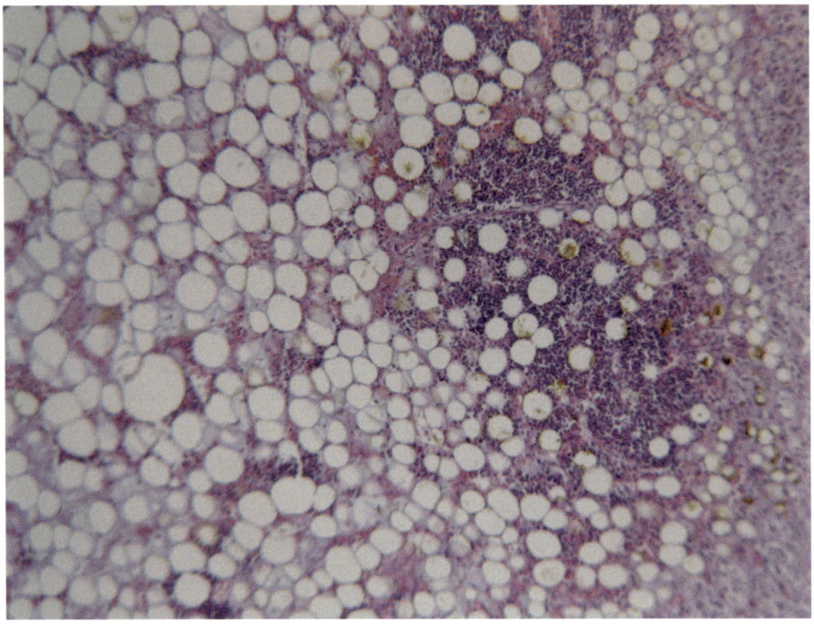

Figure 10. Microscopic appearance of myelolipoma, H&E, 120×.

higher due to the lack of diagnosis until postmortem examination; a review of autopsy cases from Australia found that 0.05% of decedents had underlying and unrecognized pheochromocytoma or paragangliomas [28].

Pheochromocytomas that grow within the adrenal medulla are the most common sympathetic ganglia-derived tumors. Conversely, paragangliomas that comprise 10–18% of all chromaffin tumors arise from the neural crest cells [29] and may derive from both parasympathetic and sympathetic ganglia. Head and neck paragangliomas originate from the parasympathetic chain (e.g. carotid body and glomus jugulotympanicus). Sympathetic-derived paragangliomas are located in the mediastinum and subdiaphragmatic regions; they are rare in comparison with parasympathetic-derived tumors.

The classic symptoms of catecholamine hypersecretion consist of headaches, sweating, and palpitations, but many patients present with sustained or paroxysmal hypertension. It has been reported, however, that pheochromocytomas associated with neurofibromatosis type 1 can present with hypotension [30]. Weight loss, myocardial infarction, hyperglycemia, panic attacks, osteolytic bone metastasis, fever, and Raynaud's phenomenon are other classical manifestations of cathecolamine-secreting paragangliomas, but only about one-third of patients demonstrate these findings [29], and many paragangliomas are not discovered until autopsy.

Sudden death due to cathecolamine-secreting tumors is very rare, and only a few isolated cases have been reported. The first reported case involves a 42-year-old woman with a 24 h history of vomiting who died suddenly. At postmortem, a 665 g pheochromocytoma was discovered at autopsy [31]. Since then, several case reports of sudden death in young and old patients harboring underlying pheochromocytomas have been described [32–36]. Interestingly, all of these patients had no history of hypertension or heart disease.

Surprisingly, large tumors, in which many of the catecholamines are metabolized internally and released mostly as by-products such as metanephrine and vanillyl mandelic acid (VMA), are more likely to be asymptomatic [29]. Patients with paragangliomas usually have classic symptoms or unusually labile hypertension that requires medical management; clinical presentation is often the main clue of a pheochromocytoma or paraganglioma, and diagnosis is usually based on the biochemical evidence of catecholamine tumor production (24-h urine metanephrines). Most updated guidelines recommend biochemical tests in symptomatic patients, patients with an adrenal incidentaloma, and patients with a hereditary risk for developing a pheochromocytoma or paraganglioma [27]. If not accompanied by any symptoms, paragangliomas, especially if located in an unusual site, can be easily missed or treated incorrectly as a benign renal or pararenal cyst. In one case report, the first manifestation of such tumor was a massive release of noradrenaline after percutaneous alcohol injection, which was performed to ablate a presumed cyst [37].

The differential diagnosis between pheochromocytoma and paraganglioma can be challenging if the tumor is located close to the upper renal pole. The first consideration is anatomic; it is well known that retroperitoneal paragangliomas can occur anywhere along the paravertebral sympathetic chain, sometimes close to the adrenal gland [38]. During the autopsy, it is important to very carefully explore the adrenal gland, or if a paraganglioma, it must be well preserved. If the tumor and adrenal gland are separate entities, and each one presents with its own capsule, pheochromocytoma can be ruled out, since it arises inside the parenchyma of the adrenal gland. A physiologic and biochemical difference between both tumors exists since pheochromocytomas and paragangliomas can secrete either adrenaline or noradrenaline. Nevertheless, pheochromocytomas produce mainly adrenaline and noradrenaline in minor quantity from the adrenal medulla, and therefore, shows a positive staining for both phenylethanolamine N-methyltransferase (the enzyme which catalyzes the synthesis of adrenaline from noradrenaline), and for dopamine-beta-hydroxylase, that is involved in both catecholamine synthetic chains. In the case of negative staining for phenylethanolamine-N-methyltransferase, and positive staining for dopamine-beta-hydroxylase, the tumor predominantly secretes noradrenaline consistent for a paraganglioma.

In cases of sudden death due to cathecholamine-secreting tumors, the external examination is often unremarkable. The decedent may be thin, but not frequently. The autopsy may reveal a tumor within the adrenal gland (pheochromocytoma) or separate from it (paraganglioma). Remarkably, paragangliomas have been found in practically every site along the sympathetic chain [38], even in the organ of Zuckerkandl [39]. Histology commonly reveals cerebral and lung congestion and edema; fibers fragmentation and many contraction bands at the myocardium (**Figure 11**).

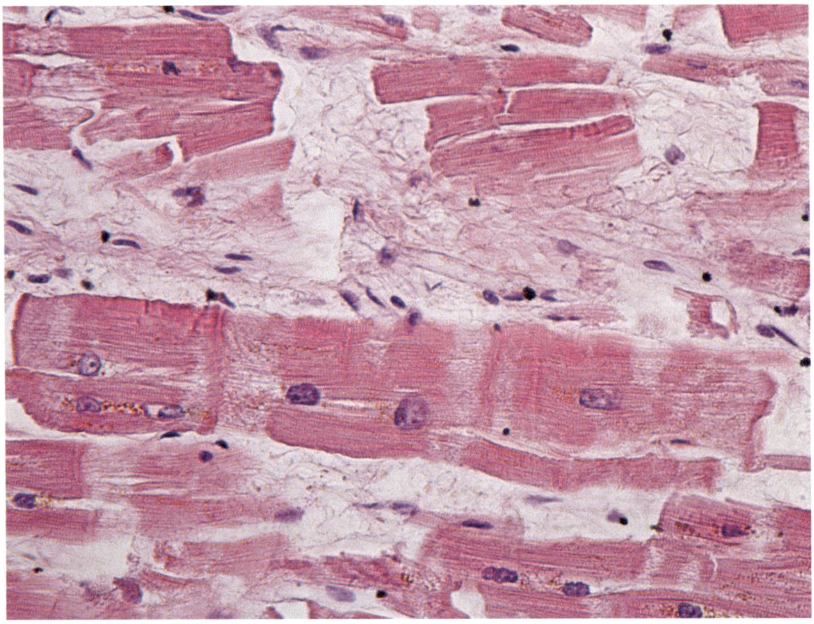

Figure 11. Myocardium, HE, 400×.

Both paragangliomas and pheochromocytomas are microscopically characterized by nests of large polygonal cells containing round and small nuclei, separated by highly vascularized fibrous septa (**Figures 12** and **13**).

Immunohistochemical examinations show chromaffin cells, chromaffin-A positive (**Figure 14**), containing enzymes involved in the synthesis of catecholamines (**Figure 15**). Chromogranin-A, which is produced only by endocrine and neuroendocrine cells, is the main soluble protein in neurosecretory granules, being co-stored and secreted with catecholamines. Another useful marker for chromaffin tumors is S100 protein (**Figure 16**), a protein specific for cells derived from the neural crest.

4.2. Embryonal neural tumors

This category encompasses neuroblastoma, ganglioneuroblastoma, and ganglioneuroma. To the authors' knowledge, there is only one case report in the literature regarding sudden death due to one of these tumors. In this sudden death of a 2-year-old child due to an unrecognized neuroblastoma, the autopsy revealed a relatively isolated adrenal mass with associated retroperitoneal hemorrhage. Microscopically, the right adrenal gland was largely composed of necrotic tissue, with only rare residual viable neoplastic cells peripherally and associated hemorrhage. Based on the gross, microscopic and microbiological findings, it was determined that the child developed rapidly lethal hemorrhagic and septic complications from an adrenal gland neuroblastoma [40].

http://dx.doi.org/10.5772/intechopen.69416

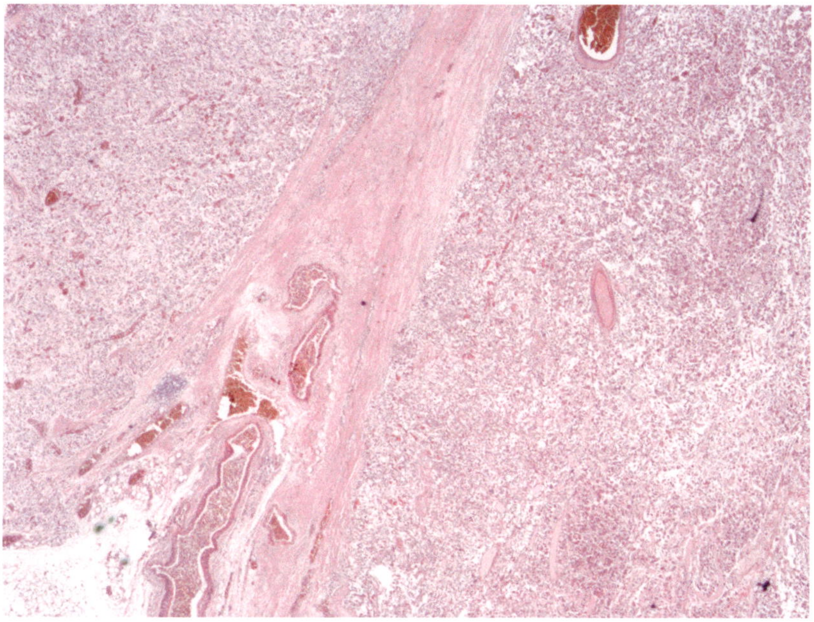

Figure 12. Paraganglioma, H&E, 20×.

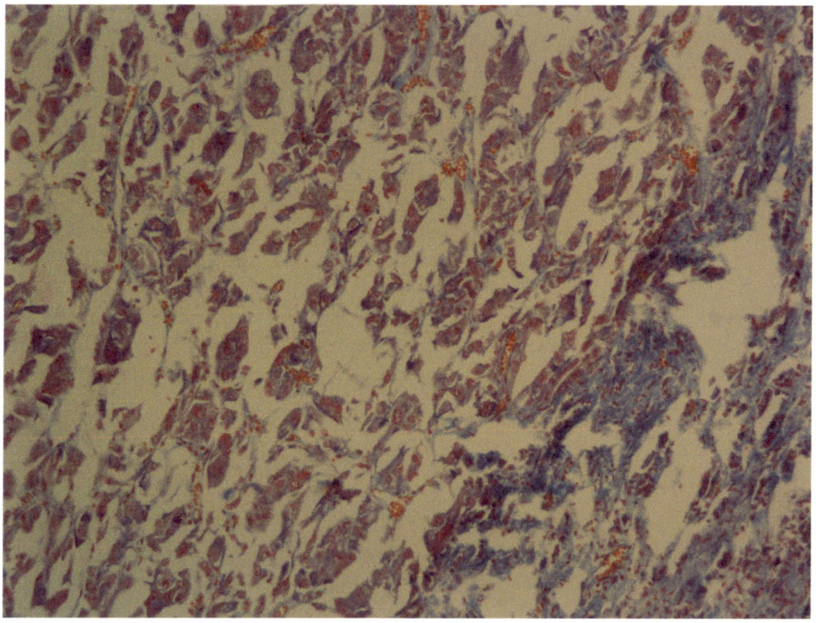

Figure 13. pheochromocytoma, H&E, 120×.

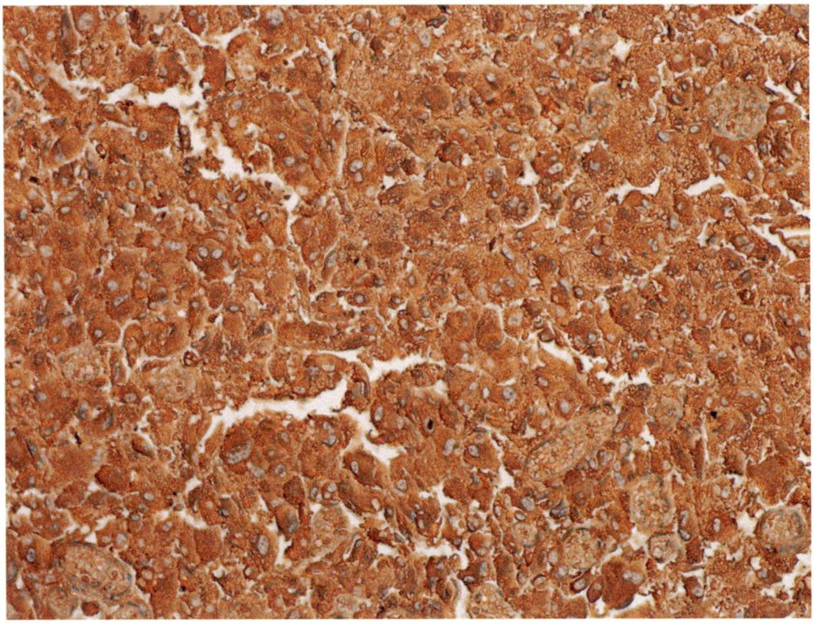

Figure 14. Antichromogranin-A, 200×. Strong positivity.

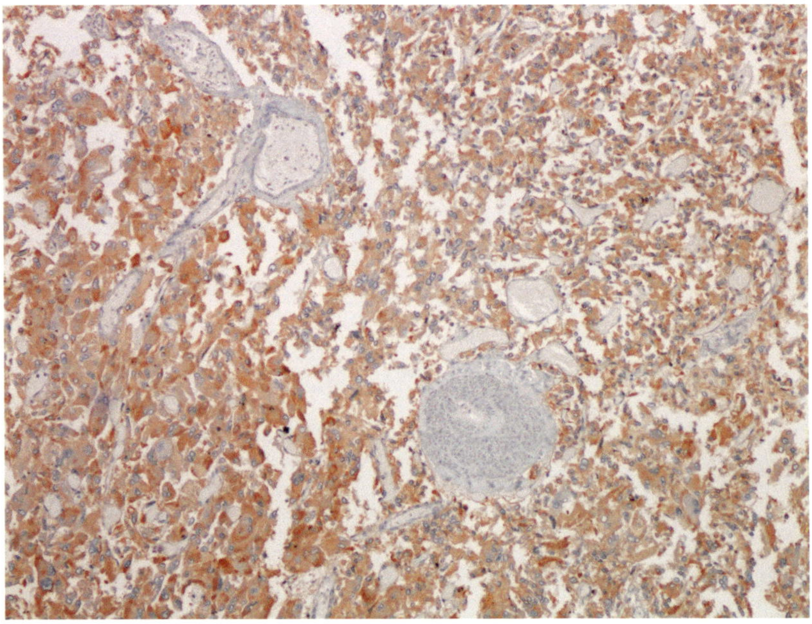

Figure 15. Antidopamine-beta-hydroxylase staining, 100×.

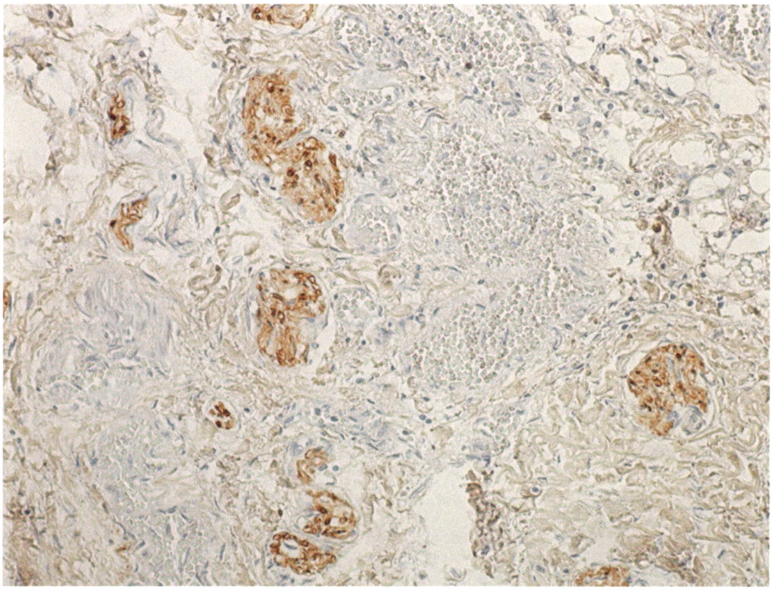

Figure 16. Anti-S100 protein staining, 100×.

5. Conclusion

This chapter provides a forensic perspective concerning sudden death due to adrenal gland diseases. Considered rare, it is seldom discussed in the literature but nevertheless encountered in clinical and forensic practice. The leading cause of sudden death related to adrenal gland disease is neuroendocrine tumors derived from chromaffin cells such as pheochromocytoma and paraganglioma, followed by adrenal hypofunction due to adrenal hemorrhage. It is imperative for both clinicians and pathologists alike to consider these diseases in daily practice. In the forensic investigations performed in cases of sudden unexpected death, especially in young individuals, a thorough examination of the adrenal glands must be performed, including macroscopic observation, as well as the microscopy using traditional stainings, such as H&E and immunohistochemistry. Conversely, if hemorrhagic in presentation, microbiologic examination of the adrenal glands should be performed in order to identify any underlying infection or sepsis.

Author details

Silvia Damiana Visonà*, Luca Tajana and Antonio Osculati

*Address all correspondence to: sd.visona@studenti.uninsubria.it

Department of Public Health, Experimental and Forensic Medicine, University of Pavia, Pavia, Italy

References

[1] Saukko P, Knight B. Knight's Forensic Pathology. 3rd ed. In: Arnold L, editor. 2004

[2] Burke MP, Opeskin K. Adrenocortical insufficiency. The American Journal of Forensic Medicine and Pathology. Mar 1999;**20**(1):60–65

[3] Govi A, Fersini F, Tsokos M. Sudden death due to acute adrenal crisis. Forensic Science, Medicine, and Pathology. Sep 2015;**11**(3):445–447

[4] Dettmeyer RB. Forensic Histopathology Fundamentals and Perspectives. Berlin Heidelberg: Springer-Verlag; 2011

[5] Al Sabri AM, Smith N, Busuttil A. Sudden death due to auto-immune Addison's disease in a 12-year-old girl. International Journal of Legal Medicine. 1997;**110**(5):278–280

[6] Clapper A, Nashelsky M, Dailey M. Evaluation of serum cortisol in the postmortem diagnosis of acute adrenal insufficiency. The American Journal of Forensic Medicine and Pathology. Jun 2008;**29**(2):181–184

[7] Palmiere C, de Froidmont S, Mangin P, Werner D, Lobrinus JA. Ketoacidosis and adrenocortical insufficiency. Journal of Forensic Sciences. Jul 2014;**59**(4):1146–1152

[8] Upadhyay J, Sudhindra P, Abraham G, Trivedi N. Tuberculosis of the adrenal gland: A case report and review of the literature of infections of the adrenal gland. International Journal of Endocrinology. 6 Aug 2014;**2014**:876037

[9] Ward S, Evans CC. Sudden death due to isolated adrenal tuberculosis. Postgraduate Medical Journal. Jul 1985;**61**(717):635–636

[10] Hofbauer LC, Heufelder AE. Endocrine implications of human immunodeficiency virus infection. Medicine. Sep 1996;**75**(5):262–278

[11] Rodrigues D, Reis M, Teixeira V, Silva-Vergara M, Filho DC, Adad S, et al. Pathologic findings in the adrenal glands of autopsied patients with acquired immunodeficiency syndrome. Pathology—Research and Practice. 2002;**198**(1):25–30

[12] Trevisan M, Matkovic U, Cusinato R, Toppo S, Palù G, Barzon L. Human cytomegalovirus productively infects adrenocortical cells and induces an early cortisol response. Journal of Cellular Physiology. Dec 2009;**221**(3):629–641

[13] Tormos LM, Schandl CA. The significance of adrenal hemorrhage: Undiagnosed Waterhouse-Friderichsen syndrome, a case series. Journal of Forensic Sciences. Jul 2013;**58**(4): 1071–1074

[14] Sahasrabudhe N, Byers R. Massive haemorrhagic adrenal metastases leading to sudden death: A case report. BMJ Case Reports [Internet]. 14 Apr 2009;**2009**. DOI: http://dx.doi.org/10.1136/bcr.06.2008.0190

[15] Michon A, Darnige L, Pouchot J, Arlet J-B. Catastrophic antiphospholipid syndrome presenting with bilateral massive adrenal haemorrhage. A case report. Joint Bone Spine. Jul 2015;**82**(4):288–289

[16] Ogino J, Toda J, Onitsuka S, Hashimoto N. Idiopathic bilateral adrenal haemorrhage related to acute adrenal insufficiency. BMJ Case Reports [Internet]. 31 May 2013;**2013**. DOI: http://dx.doi.org/10.1136/bcr-2013-009626

[17] McGowan-Smyth S. Bilateral adrenal haemorrhage leading to adrenal crisis. BMJ Case Reports [Internet]. 26 Jun 2014;**2014**. DOI: http://dx.doi.org/10.1136/bcr-2014-204225

[18] Lefevre N, Delaunay L, Hingot JL, Bonnet F. Bilateral massive adrenal haemorrhage complicating anaphylactic shock: A case report. Intensive Care Medicine. May 1996;**22**(5): 447–449

[19] Vella A, Nippoldt TB, Morris JC 3rd. Adrenal hemorrhage: A 25-year experience at the Mayo clinic. Mayo Clinic Proceedings. Feb 2001;**76**(2):161–168

[20] Jennewein C, Tran N, Kanczkowski W, Heerdegen L, Kantharajah A, Dröse S, et al. Mortality of septic mice strongly correlates with adrenal gland inflammation. Critical Care Medicine. Apr 2016;**44**(4):e190-e199

[21] Fox B. Disseminated intravascular coagulation and the Waterhouse-Friderichsen syndrome. Archives of Disease in Childhood. Oct 1971;**46**(249):680–685

[22] Graversen D, Vestergaard P, Stochholm K, Gravholt CH, Jørgensen JOL. Mortality in Cushing's syndrome: A systematic review and meta-analysis. European Journal of Internal Medicine. Apr 2012;**23**(3):278–282

[23] Gkourogianni A, Lodish MB, Zilbermint M, Lyssikatos C, Belyavskaya E, Keil MF, et al. Death in pediatric Cushing syndrome is uncommon but still occurs. European Journal of Pediatrics. Apr 2015;**174**(4):501–507

[24] Gerson SN, Miclat R. Cushing disease presenting as atypical psychosis followed by sudden death. The Canadian Journal of Psychiatry. Apr 1985;**30**(3):223–224

[25] Scott BD, Friday KJ. Cushing's syndrome presenting as sudden death. American Heart Journal. Feb 1988;**115**(2):487–488

[26] Yildiz L, Akpolat I, Erzurumlu K, Aydin O, Kandemir B. Giant adrenal myelolipoma: Case report and review of the literature. Pathology International. Jun 2000;**50**(6):502–504

[27] Lee JA, Duh Q-Y. Sporadic paraganglioma. World Journal of Surgery. May 2008;**32**(5):683–687

[28] Abadin SS, Ayala-Ramirez M, Jimenez C, Dickson PV, Liang Y, Lazar AJ, et al. Impact of surgical resection for subdiaphragmatic paragangliomas. World Journal of Surgery. Mar 2014;**38**(3):733–741

[29] Chen H, Sippel RS, O'Dorisio MS, Vinik AI, Lloyd RV, Pacak K, et al. The North American neuroendocrine tumor society consensus guideline for the diagnosis and management of neuroendocrine tumors: Pheochromocytoma, paraganglioma, and medullary thyroid cancer. Pancreas. Aug 2010;**39**(6):775–783

[30] Cecchi R, Frati P, Capri O, Cipolloni L. A rare case of sudden death due to hypotension during cesarean section in a woman suffering from pheochromocytoma and neurofibromatosis. Journal of Forensic Sciences. Nov 2013;**58**(6):1636–1639

[31] Vallance WB. Sudden death from an asymptomatic phaeochromocytoma. British Medical Journal. 23 Mar 1957;**1**(5020):686–687

[32] Verzeletti A, Amariti ML. Sudden death from an asymptomatic phaeochromocytoma: A case report. Journal of Forensic and Legal Medicine. May 2011;**18**(4):180–181

[33] Preuss J, Woenckhaus C, Schwesinger G, Madea B. Non-diagnosed pheochromocytoma as a cause of sudden death in a 49-year-old man: A case report with medico-legal implications. Forensic Science International. 27 Jan 2006;**156**(2-3):223–228

[34] Primhak RA, Spicer RD, Variend S. Sudden death after minor abdominal trauma: An unusual presentation of phaeochromocytoma. British Medical Journal. 11 Jan 1986;**292**(6513):95–96

[35] Chiu C-C, Chen Y-C, Teng T-H, Yang L-H, Chen Y-P, Siao F-Y. Sudden cardiac arrest after minor abdominal trauma: A successful resuscitation in a patient with haemorrhagic phaeochromocytoma. Resuscitation. Nov 2009;**80**(11):1323–1324

[36] Osculati A, Motta M. Morte improvvisa associata a feocromocitoma. Medicina Legale Quaderni Camerti. 1999; anno XXI

[37] Andrello L, Visonà SD, Osculati A. A case of sudden death after ultrasound-guided percutaneous alcohol injection of a paraganglioma mis-diagnosed as a peri-renal cyst. Forensic Science International. Aug 2015;**253**:e20-e24

[38] Rosai J. Rosai and Ackerman's Surgical Pathology. Vol. 1. Mosby, St. Louis, MO, USA, 2004

[39] Sperry K, Smialek JE. Sudden death due to a paraganglioma of the organs of Zuckerkandl. The American Journal of Forensic Medicine and Pathology. Mar 1986;**7**(1):23–29

[40] Park KU, Prahlow JA. Sudden death due to adrenal neuroblastoma: Child abuse mimic? Forensic Science, Medicine, and Pathology. Mar 2011;**7**(1):47–52